D1613537

MANAGING CARE, NOT DOLLARS

The Continuum of Mental Health Services

MANAGING CARE, NOT DOLLARS

The Continuum of Mental Health Services

Edited by

Robert K. Schreter, M.D.
Steven S. Sharfstein, M.D., M.P.A.
Carol A. Schreter, M.S.W., Ph.D.

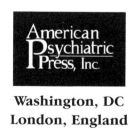

American Psychiatric Press, Inc.

Washington, DC
London, England

Note: The authors have worked to ensure that all information in this book concerning drug dosages, schedules, and routes of administration is accurate as of the time of publication and consistent with standards set by the U.S. Food and Drug Administration and the general medical community. As medical research and practice advance, however, therapeutic standards may change. For this reason and because human and mechanical errors sometimes occur, we recommend that readers follow the advice of a physician who is directly involved in their care or the care of a member of their family.

Books published by the American Psychiatric Press, Inc., represent the views and opinions of the individual authors and do not necessarily represent the policies and opinions of the Press or the American Psychiatric Association.

Copyright © 1997 American Psychiatric Press, Inc.
ALL RIGHTS RESERVED
Manufactured in the United States of America on acid-free paper
00 99 98 97   4 3 2 1

American Psychiatric Press, Inc.
1400 K Street, N.W., Washington, DC   20005

Library of Congress Cataloging-in-Publication Data
Managing care, not dollars : the continuum of mental health services /
    edited by Robert K. Schreter, Steven S. Sharfstein, Carol A.
    Schreter.
        p.   cm.
    Includes bibliographical references and index.
    ISBN 0-88048-855-7 (cloth : alk. paper)
    1. Mental health services—Administration.   2. Managed mental
health care.   3. Mental health services—Finance.   I. Schreter,
Robert K., 1945–   . II. Sharfstein, Steven S. (Steven Samuel),
1942–   . III. Schreter, Carol A., 1947–   .
    [DNLM: 1. Mental Health Services—organization & administration—
United States.   2. Managed Care Programs—organization &
administration—United States.   3. Continuity of Patient Care—
economics—United States.   WM 30 M2665 1997]
RA790.5.M29   1997
362.2′068—dc20
DNLM/DLC
for Library of Congress   96-24028
                                                                        CIP

British Library Cataloguing in Publication Data
A CIP record is available from the British Library.

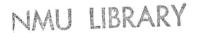

CONTENTS

SECTION 1

Components of the Continuum

SECTION II

Using the Continuum for Children,
Adolescents, and the Elderly

Planning and Administering the Continuum

SECTION IV

Public Policy Issues and the Continuum

SECTION V

Conclusion

CONTRIBUTORS

Richard Altman, M.S.W.
Deputy Executive Vice President, Jewish Child Care Association of New York; Team Leader, Council on Accreditation, Child Welfare League of America, New York, New York

Bernard S. Arons, M.D.
Director, Center for Mental Health Services, Substance Abuse and Mental Health Services Administration, Rockville, Maryland

Alan A. Axelson, M.D.
Medical Director and Chief Executive Officer, InterCare Behavioral Health Systems, Pittsburgh, Pennsylvania; Member and Past Chairman, Task Force on Managed Care, American Academy of Child and Adolescent Psychiatry, Washington, D.C.

John Bartlett, M.D., M.P.H.
Executive Vice President, Quality Improvement, Magellan Health Services, Atlanta, Georgia

Simon H. Budman, Ph.D.
Director of Mental Health Training, Harvard Community Health Plan, Boston, Massachusetts; President and Founder, Innovative Training Systems, Inc., Newton, Massachusetts

Richard D. Budson, M.D.
Associate Clinical Professor of Psychiatry, Harvard Medical School, Boston, Massachusetts; Attending Psychiatrist, McLean Hospital, Belmont, Massachusetts

Dorothy E. Dugger, M.D.
President, Dugger Consulting, Chester Springs, Pennsylvania; Clinical Associate Professor of Psychiatry, Temple University Medical School, Philadelphia, Pennsylvania

David Fassler, M.D.
President, Choate Health Systems, Inc., Woburn, Massachusetts; Clinical Director, Otter Creek Associates, Burlington, Vermont

Paul Jay Fink, M.D.
Associate Vice President, Albert Einstein Health Care Network; Director, Einstein Center for the Study of Violence, Belmont Center for Comprehensive Treatment, Philadelphia, Pennsylvania

Laurie M. Flynn
Executive Director, National Alliance for the Mentally Ill (NAMI), Arlington, Virginia

Robert J. Fox, J.D.
Director of Planning, Continuum Behavioral Healthcare, Park Ridge, New Jersey

Richard J. Frances, M.D.
Chairman, Department of Psychiatry, Hackensack University Medical Center, Hackensack, New Jersey; Professor of Clinical Psychiatry, Department of Psychiatry, University of Medicine and Dentistry of New Jersey–New Jersey Medical School, Newark

Ronald D. Geraty, M.D.
President and CEO, Continuum Behavioral Healthcare Corporation; Executive Vice President, Merit Behavioral Care Corporation, Park Ridge, New Jersey

Gail Hanson-Mayer, R.N., C.S., M.P.H.
Senior Vice President, Operations, Choate Health Management, Inc., Stoneham, Massachusetts

Terri Hubbard, M.S., L.M.H.C.
Director, Psychiatric Emergency Services, Choate Health Management, Inc., Stoneham, Massachusetts

Ira Kaufman, M.S.W.
Director of Foster Home Division, Jewish Child Care Association of New York, New York

John J. Kent Jr., J.D.
Executive Vice President and Chief Operating Officer, Sheppard and Enoch Pratt Health System, Baltimore, Maryland

Laurel J. Kiser, Ph.D., M.B.A.
Executive Director, Child and Adolescent Partial Hospitalization Programs, and Professor, Department of Psychiatry, University of Tennessee College of Medicine, Memphis

Arthur Lazarus, M.D.
Medical Director, Northwestern Institute, Fort Washington, Pennsylvania; Clinical Associate Professor of Psychiatry, Temple University Hospital, Philadelphia, Pennsylvania

Paul R. McCarthy, Ph.D.
Vice President, Quality Improvement and Outcomes Management, Green Spring Health Services, Columbia, Maryland

Samuel Moy, Ph.D.
President, Positive Alternatives to Hospitalization (PATH) Professional Corporation; Vice President of Clinical Services, PATHwise Behavioral Health, Inc., Farmington, Connecticut

H. Edmund Pigott, Ph.D.
President, PATHware, Inc., Kensington, Connecticut

David B. Pruitt, M.D.
Director, Division of Child and Adolescent Psychiatry, and Professor, Department of Psychiatry, University of Tennessee College of Medicine, Memphis

Robert P. Roca, M.D., M.P.H.
Director, Geriatric Services, The Sheppard and Enoch Pratt Health System; Associate Professor of Psychiatry, The Johns Hopkins University School of Medicine, Baltimore, Maryland

Alvin A. Rosenfeld, M.D.
Former Director, Psychiatric Services, Jewish Child Care Association of New York, New York; Co-Chair, Foster Care and Adoption Committee, American Academy of Child and Adolescent Psychiatry, Washington, D.C.; private practice in psychiatry, and consultant, New York City, New York, and Greenwich, Connecticut

Donald R. Ross, M.D.
Director, Division of Education and Residency Training, Sheppard and Enoch Pratt Health System, Baltimore, Maryland

Carol A. Schreter, M.S.W., Ph.D.
Authors' editor and freelance writer on health and aging, Baltimore, Maryland

Robert K. Schreter, M.D.
Medical Director, Sheppard Pratt Health Plan; Assistant Professor of Psychiatry, Johns Hopkins School of Medicine, Baltimore, Maryland

Steven S. Sharfstein, M.D., M.P.A.
Medical Director and CEO, The Sheppard and Enoch Pratt Health System; Clinical Professor of Psychiatry, University of Maryland Medical School, Baltimore, Maryland

William E. Stone, M.D.
Medical Director, Health Management Strategies International, Alexandria, Virginia; former Gladys and R. Lee Kempner Professor of Child and Adolescent Psychiatry, University of Texas Medical Branch, Galveston

Sandra Raynes Weiss
Special Assistant to the Administrator, Substance Abuse and Mental Health Services Administration, Rockville, Maryland

Judith H. Wiegand, M.A.
Administrative Director, Planning/Marketing/Managed Care, Hackettstown Community Hospital, Hackettstown, New Jersey

Evelyn Wilson, M.S.W.
Supervisor, Addiction Treatment Center and the Adolescent Drug and Alcohol Prevention and Treatment Program (ADAPT), Hackensack University Medical Center, Hackensack, New Jersey

Robert Wisner-Carlson, M.D.
Senior Psychiatrist/Service Chief, Short-Term/Managed Care Unit, The Sheppard and Enoch Pratt Health System, Baltimore, Maryland

1 Managing Care, Not Dollars

Robert K. Schreter, M.D.
Steven S. Sharfstein, M.D., M.P.A.
Carol A. Schreter, M.S.W., Ph.D.

By 1994, the total cost of health care in the United States approached $900 billion annually. This is fueling a demand for cost containment, evidence of clinical effectiveness, and guaranteed coverage for all Americans. Cost has become a critical factor in the delivery of health and mental health services. Fearful that mental health care in particular will become unaffordable, both government and industry will likely turn to some form of global budgeting.

In *Allies and Adversaries: The Impact of Managed Care on Mental Health Services* (Schreter et al. 1994), we, as editors, focused on the question What has been the impact of managed care on mental health services? Since then, many clinicians seem to have grudgingly come to accept the inevitability of managed care and cost controls.

Today's most frequently asked question is, How can we make the management of care work for patients and clinicians? Too many people seem to think that the answer lies in playing with

1

the dollars. But we, the editors, believe the answer lies rather in advances in treatment, developing a continuum of care, and effectively linking the various components into a coherent system.

The concept of the continuum of care with multiple components is not a new idea. It derives from community mental health principles and ideas developed in the 1960s as a means to provide continuity of care, a requirement in the early regulations for community mental health centers. Throughout the last two decades, the public mental health delivery system has moved services out of the hospital into the community, developed alternatives for patients with serious long-term mental illness and substance abuse, and diversified the treatment into a range of choices for patients and providers. The movement toward managed care and capitation to reduce costs, with its profound impact on access and quality, provides the next stage for developing the continuum concept. The continuum is now serving patients with private health insurance.

Until recently, the highest-intensity services were provided only at the highest level of care—at the psychiatric hospital. However, intensity of service and location can be uncoupled. For instance, the treatment of acute psychosis and detoxification from substances of abuse is no longer automatically seen as an inpatient procedure. Newer medications with less compromising side effects are reducing symptoms. Patients can now be treated outside of the hospital, at lower levels of care.

In the early years, lower levels of care were utilized only as a "step down" for patients making the transition from full-time hospital care to home. More recently, lower levels of care are gaining importance as hospital diversion techniques. Some involve direct but limited contact with a mental health facility: partial hospital, day and evening hospitals, residential treatment centers, and halfway houses. Other services are community based, such as home-based interventions, emergency crisis services, school-based programs, and drop-in centers. Clinicians are now also using their offices for a greater variety of outpatient services, including individual, couple, family and group psychotherapies, rehabilitation services, and case management of high-risk/high-cost patients.

This array of interventions is often dubbed a *continuum.* Now such interventions are valued for their cost savings when compared with acute hospital days. In the future, these services will likely be important because they offer special clinical advantages.

Midpoint clinical services along this continuum are not unfamiliar to most clinicians, but they are not readily available in each locale. This is in part because payers for care—government, industry, and third-party insurers—have avoided reimbursement for these services. This is changing, especially with prospective payment and capitated care, where a contract provides a fixed sum per person covered. We can anticipate payment for those services that work and make economic sense. With prospective payment, clinicians now have the opportunity to develop innovative programs. We should anticipate the need for outcomes data that prove that these newer services are clinically effective.

In Section I, "Components of the Continuum," the chapter authors describe state-of-the-art programs with a level of precision not previously available. Clinical innovators discuss who is best served by each option and how to develop, staff, and run each program.

In Section II, "Using the Continuum for Children, Adolescents, and the Elderly," the chapter authors recognize that the young and old have special needs. For these populations, there may need to be a parallel continuum with some additional components to take advantage of existing age-specific settings such as the school and nursing home.

In Section III, "Planning and Administering the Continuum," the chapter authors provide decision-making tools for managers. They recognize that the continuum requires a new infrastructure and large-scale information systems. How does an existing program—an academic department, a hospital, a clinical group, or a community mental health center—adapt, survive, and grow in this new era? Sharfstein and Kent (Chapter 18) describe how one institution downsized the hospital and upsized the continuum components.

In Section IV, "Public Policy Issues and the Continuum," Arons and Weiss (Chapter 20) explore how the public community mental health centers learned to expand the continuum for people with severe and persistent mental illness. For them to regain and maintain optimal function, the continuum must provide nonmedical supports, including supervision, food, and shelter. From the family viewpoint, Flynn (Chapter 21) further elongates the continuum by describing the critical role of family and nonmedical community resources. The authors of both chapters seem to argue that the public sector evolution should be used now to inform the private sector revolution in mental health care.

Even at this early stage in the developing continuum of care, it is possible to identify a set of emerging principles that guide the continuum's development. From the insurer's viewpoint, there seem to be two overriding principles:

1. *Keep a population-based perspective.* The clinician's responsibility has been expanded beyond the current patient to include all potential patients who have not yet presented for care. Under capitation and global budgeting, clinicians must shepherd limited resources to ensure maximum benefit for the larger society.
2. *Follow the principle of parsimony.* Treat patients with the least expensive, least intensive treatment alternative at the lowest level of care that is adequate to return the patient to health and function.

To accomplish these overriding goals, the managed care industry seems to be expecting clinicians to follow other principles, such as those presented next. As described in Chapters 20 and 21, some of the principles that guide the development of the continuum grew out of the public community mental health center movement or reflect the consumer view.

Be Innovative With Time, Treatment Setting, and Therapeutic Modalities

The use of group rather than individual treatments, educational rather than insight-oriented approaches, and time-sensitive episodic care instead of continuous care is encouraged. Hospitalization is indicated only when no other suitable treatments are available.

Treatment Should Be Flexible, Individualized, and Goal Oriented

Clinicians are encouraged to identify individualized treatment goals, initiate treatment specific to the presenting problem, and conclude this episode of care as soon as treatment goals have been attained. Programs of fixed length, such as 28-day drug and alcohol programs or programs in which the patients course through the program based on arbitrarily determined steps, are no longer reimbursable by medical insurance.

Set Up Comprehensive Systems of Care

The scope and array of services must be great enough to address the needs of all patients and the needs of one patient at different times in his or her illness. It must provide an adequate range of choices as patients move from acute inpatient or intermediate care into less intensive community-based services.

Make Care Available and Accessible

Patients must be able to enter and utilize the services with ease. Barriers to care such as gatekeeping and cost must be kept to a bare minimum.

Provide Clinical Care as Close to Home and the Patient's Support Systems as Possible

Providing clinical care as close to home and the patient's support systems as possible increases diagnostic precision, encourages family support, and facilitates return to home, school, and workplace. Stigma must be minimized. Work, housing, leisure programs, and community supports should be integrated into the patient's overall treatment and rehabilitation plan.

Be Consumer Oriented When Designing Systems

Patients and their families must have substantial roles in determining program design and in the monitoring of quality, outcome, and compliance. In the future, many services will be provided by nonprofessionals, at points beyond the medical continuum of care.

Hold Providers and Systems of Care Accountable for Their Care

Quality standards must be monitored. Use valid and reliable outcome measures, including clinical, social, and financial outcomes for continuous quality improvement.

Integrated Systems of Care Should Be Our Goal

The systems must minimize the impact of fragmentation that results from a multiplicity of treatment sites, providers, and payers. Careful attention must be paid to the linkages—the flow of patients and information over time, space, and systems.

Case Management Services Are an Increasingly Important Part of Treatment

To ensure a patient's optimal use of treatment, a case manager follows an individual patient over time, talking with the patient's various providers and support systems, sometimes interacting with the patient as well.

The Shift Toward a Strong Interdisciplinary Approach to Care Is Helpful

Teams of clinicians who can contribute different areas of expertise may increase clinical efficiency in getting patients back to home, work, and community.

Conclusion

Overall, this book is a how-to manual, *a guide to setting up and using the emerging continuum of care.* The editors believe that our existing psychiatric institutions can no longer survive as isolated programs providing a single service. Instead, the institutions will need to provide the full range of services to large numbers of patients, and perhaps share in the insurance risk.

It now seems that clinicians' survival and patients' well-being will depend on our creativity, on each community's ability to develop an effective continuum of mental health services.

Reference

Schreter RK, Sharfstein SS, Schreter CA (eds): Allies and Adversaries: The Impact of Managed Care on Mental Health Services. Washington, DC, American Psychiatric Press, 1994

I

Components of
the Continuum

2 Office-Based Services

Robert K. Schreter, M.D.
Simon H. Budman, Ph.D.

Office-based care no longer connotes the solo practitioner working in relative isolation who sees patients weekly at a private office. The following case illustrates how office-based practice now involves time-effective treatment, the use of different levels of clinical resources, case consultation, and the delivery of services through a system of care.

When Valerie was first seen, she was 16 years old and had dropped out of high school. Her parents were separated for more than 9 years. Valerie had lived for a year with her father, Mr. S, a rigid and angry man, who had taken her into his home after she had run away from her mother, who lived in a distant state. The patient's mother (who was never seen by the therapist) appeared to be, based on description, an extremely disturbed, paranoid schizophrenic person, who at the time retained custody of Valerie's younger 8-year-old sister, Amanda. Shortly after Valerie ran away, Valerie's mother moved back to the Boston area with Amanda.

Mr. S brought Valerie in for treatment because she "could not" get herself ready for school and exhibited strange, compulsive rituals related to washing and taking showers for several hours each morning. These rituals (e.g., needing to leave soap on her skin in the shower for at least 45 minutes before washing it off) interfered with her schooling, work, and social interactions. Shortly after the therapist initially met with Valerie, he referred her to a partial hospitalization program associated with the group practice where she was being treated. Valerie spent 18 days, spread over about 6 weeks, in the partial hospitalization program. During her partial hospitalization stay, she was evaluated for medication and began to take fluoxetine hydrochloride and lithium. The medication was useful to her, although some of the compulsive behavior remained problematic.

On discharge, Valerie began to see her outpatient therapist on a weekly basis, but within a month, she had dropped out of treatment and stopped her medication. Her symptoms returned, and she regressed significantly. In a team clinical meeting, her clinician was urged to ask Valerie and her father to come in together for a consultation session with several of the team clinicians and her primary clinician present. A number of important factors that were adversely affecting the treatment came to light. One was that Valerie was having a difficult time feeling comfortable with her therapist. (She indicated that she had a hard time trusting a woman because she identified the therapist too closely with her mother.) Valerie was switched to a male therapist on the team. From that time forward, she was seen by this therapist with her father present. It became clear to the team that the father could not really allow her to see a therapist on her own and felt too threatened by this. Valerie and her father continued in family therapy, and she also saw a psychopharmacologist periodically. Valerie and her father were seen approximately every 6–7 weeks over the next 2 years. The sessions included a great deal of work on helping Valerie and her father work out important aspects of their relationship, such as Valerie's discomfort with her father's constant need to control all aspects of her behavior and his unwill-

ingness at times to pay for her medications. From Mr. S's
point of view, he felt that Valerie was irresponsible and unwilling to work, go to school, get a "better" group of
friends, and so on. Most sessions included "homework" for
both Mr. S and Valerie. Although the course of the treatment
was rocky and difficult, 2 years after treatment began
Valerie was able to get her general equivalency diploma and
has since entered college and successfully completed her
freshman year.

There were several foci in working with Valerie. First, it was
clearly important for her to remain on her medications and to
find ways to help her be more compliant with continuing on
these. Second, her father needed to be integrated into the treatment process because he was in a position that could sabotage
the work that Valerie was doing. It was important to enlist him
in the process. Finally, other resources needed to be pulled into
Valerie's case. Based on a referral to her state rehabilitation services, she was able to get employment testing and some prelimi-
nary training services through a rehabilitation program.

Time-Effective Therapy: A Clinical Model for the Continuum of Care

For many years, the treatment of choice for both inpatient and
outpatient clinicians was long-term care. Outpatient treatment,
on average, has never been very long. However, in the minds of
many therapists, it was ideally seen as long term and open
ended. Most of the briefer treatment that took place was un-
planned and short term by default rather than by design (for a
discussion, see Budman and Gurman 1988).

With the rise of managed care, the pendulum has swung.
Some managed behavioral health care companies press providers to treat patients with severe and chronic disorders within
therapies of five to eight weekly visits. There has been a whole-
sale rush toward short-term, "solution-oriented" therapies.

Although there are many useful elements to these models, their explosive growth has taken place without systematic research or empirical support. However, some managed care companies take the blanket position espoused by more radical solution-oriented brief therapists that almost all patients can be seen in very short-term, time-limited treatments. These care managers seem to neglect or are unaware of extensive bodies of longitudinal epidemiological data indicating the chronic and relapsing nature of certain problems such as major depression, substance abuse, and personality disorders. For the most part, with such disorders, useful treatment does not guarantee future success. Even imagining that such prophylaxis could occur as a result of psychotherapy is naive and akin to assuming that catching the flu will prevent you from getting a different strain of the flu next year, or keep you from getting heart disease or appendicitis.

Everyone cannot be cured forever in 1–2 months of treatment, nor does everyone need to be treated in years of ongoing individual therapy. A model of treatment that is far more congruent with both clinical and economic realities is the time-effective therapy model described by Budman and Gurman (1988). The key conceptual elements of this model as summarized by Budman (1994) are as follows.

Parsimony and Small Changes Are More Important Than "Cure"

If one can use a parsimonious, "minimalist" intervention to achieve even a small change, this may have major implications for the individual, couple, or family. This is due to a process described by chaos theory experts—chaologists—as a feedback process (Briggs and Peat 1989). Such feedback processes in nature are self-amplifying. Small changes can lead to big differences.

A Population-Based Perspective Is Maintained

Most clinicians will find themselves participating in systems that demand that they not only treat individuals, couples, or families, but also that they assume responsibility for a population of patients.

Viewing Patients From an Adult Developmental Perspective Is Encouraged

This perspective assumes that people are already in the process of change when they come to see us. Adults continue to change throughout the life cycle and are not to be viewed as lacking an internal momentum toward improvement. A view of change coming from analytic thinking has been that people basically stop making many transformations after young adulthood. The time-effective model holds that change persists throughout the life span. Because we are all continually changing, there is an increased possibility for patients to move forward with and improve their lives.

Patient Strengths and Resources Should Be Emphasized

In the past, many treatment models were strongly oriented toward patient pathology. With advances in solution-oriented treatments (e.g., DeShazer 1992) and cognitive-behavioral approaches (e.g., Beck et al. 1979), patients' strengths are being increasingly emphasized.

Most Changes Occur Between Sessions

There are many more hours between therapy sessions than within sessions. The therapist needs to find ways to help the patient "carry" the therapy/therapist outside of therapy sessions. Homework assignments and between-session tasks are very important elements of time-effective treatment and allow the work to continue outside the consultation room.

Change Is Not a Linear Process

Countless significant processes in nature tend not to be uniform, smooth, or linear. Although patient change processes in psychotherapy are often discussed as if they were gradual and linear, this is rarely the case. Often, there are extended periods for the patient during which little or nothing appears to be happening (on the surface). Then suddenly "something clicks," and the patient can act and think in ways that he or she could not or did not do previously. It appears that change processes are cumulative and that patients take different things from different episodes of therapy. It may seem to the therapist that a particular episode of treatment was not useful or helpful to the patient. It is only years later, with additional episodes of treatment and with certain life events occurring, that the patient is able make use of the earlier input.

Fiscal and Resource Allocation Issues Are Critically Important in Time-Effective Therapy

For the most part, therapists tend not to operate in time-effective ways by choice (at least initially). A high degree of thoughtful organization and planning is required for a clinician to manage a caseload in ways that are time effective. For an organization, moving clinicians in a direction that is time sensitive may engender conflict within the organizational culture and may also incur training and reorganization costs (Bennett 1993; Budman and Armstrong 1992).

Psychotherapy Is Viewed as Being for Better or for Worse

Psychotherapy, like any other mental or physical treatment, can have negative side effects. There are people who suffer from a virtual "addiction" to psychotherapy. These people feel themselves unable to live without ongoing treatment. For this population, Budman and Gurman (1988) advocated "treatment-free periods." Such periods outside mental health therapy may allow people to consolidate what they have learned.

Supporting Systems: A Key Aspect of Becoming Time Effective

Clinicians can operate more time-effectively if systems are in place that reinforce the delivery of such treatment. There are several clinical system elements that can encourage and support the delivery of time-effective care.

An Extensive Program of Group Psychotherapy

It is critically important that a program of time-effective care include an extensive outpatient group treatment program. Some of these groups may be time-limited and short-term interactional or psychoeducational and others longer term and/or open ended. Longer-term groups, especially interpersonal/interactional groups, appear to be a very useful modality for patients with severe personality disorders. Such a group program will allow clinicians to have options for patients that are time effective and efficient. Furthermore, the research data seem to support the efficacy of group treatment when compared with individual treatment.

Institutional Flexibility Regarding Management of Schedules

An important component of time-effective outpatient treatment is the flexible use of time (Budman 1994; Budman and Gurman 1988). If therapists are locked in to hourly sessions administratively or because of theoretical orientation must maintain fixed and rigid scheduling of patients (e.g., weekly, hour-long sessions), time-effective therapy will not take place.

Clinician-Friendly Record Keeping and Paperwork

Clinicians cannot be seeing patients in efficient ways if they are bogged down with endless, burdensome paperwork. Paperwork demands need to be carefully assessed, and others need to do whatever possible so that the clinician can work with patients rather than fill out an endless number of forms. Some paperwork could be completed by the patient him- or herself or with the assistance of nonclinical staff.

Clinician Incentives for Efficiency and Effectiveness

It is critically important to clarify the direction in which incentives within the system encourage the clinicians to move. Are there incentives for keeping the patient in weekly treatment for an extended period? (For example, will it be difficult to fill a time slot if I see my patients *too* efficiently?) Are there incentives for seeing many new patients but few incentives for maintaining patient satisfaction? Does the therapist have any input or knowledge regarding the outcomes of his or her patients? Do incentives move the therapist toward getting involved with more and more nonclinical meetings? The list could go on. If you wish to organize a time-effective treatment service, you must be clear about what the systemic incentives are and in which directions these encourage clinicians to go.

Support of Clinician Time-Efficiency With Training and Consultation

It is unlikely that clinicians can practice time-effective therapy without strong supports in the areas of training and consultation. As Budman and Armstrong (1992) wrote, such training is a crucial part of the delivery of this mode of care. Most mental health clinicians have not been adequately prepared for practicing in a time-effective manner. Without adequate training and ongoing clinical input, it is most difficult to practice in this way. This is particularly true because time-effective treatment requires great flexibility and familiarity with a wide variety of theoretical and intervention approaches.

Belief "at the Top" That
Time-Effective Therapy Works

If clinicians believe that brief treatment is a ruse to enable a group of mental health entrepreneurs to make money, many negative consequences follow. The clinicians may feel that the agency or organization they are working for is a self-serving concern, with no real desire to offer high-quality care. Therapists will feel demoralized and assume they must fight the system for the patient to get what he or she deserves. The self-esteem and creativity of staff will fall, and people will try to find ways to bide their time. Staff will begin to feel angry with their patients because each new patient represents another "problem" to be gotten rid of as soon as possible. Clinician managers in a time-effective system ideally should be practicing, committed, time-effective therapists who believe in the value and usefulness of such care. They should also understand the problems of their staff clinicians and the ways in which the delivery of clinical care in the model differ from other types of clinical delivery systems.

Managed Care: Impetus for Change

The increasing popularity of time-effective therapies is directly related to the growth of managed care. An estimated 75% of employees at moderate size to large American businesses now receive managed mental health services (England 1994). This number can be expected to approach 100% in the near future. Solo practice and fee-for-service reimbursement are rapidly disappearing. Under managed competition, accountable health plans will direct the care of vast numbers of "covered lives" into integrated health systems.

Payers now favor outpatient care over inpatient services because of the apparent cost advantage. Only a decade ago, 66% of the health care dollar went to pay for inpatient services. Today, the ratio of inpatient to outpatient costs is being reversed. An estimated 50%–60% of each dollar is now directed to outpatient care.

New Criteria Favor Office-Based Services

Current criteria make office-based services the treatment of choice for all situations where there are not specific contraindications. This greatly expands the spectrum of disorders and the severity of symptoms that are being treated at this level of care.

Previously, certain Axis I diagnoses or specific signs and symptoms, such as suicidal ideation, were seen as an automatic indicator for referral to inpatient care. Instead of relying on automatic indicators, triage clinicians are beginning to asses clinical presentations in terms of three independent variables: 1) severity of symptoms, 2) intensity of needed service, and 3) available options along a continuum of care. Uncoupling these factors permits the independent evaluation of each. Clinicians will find this greatly expands the range of treatment options and the number of patients referred for outpatient services and office-based services.

Emergence of Behavioral Group Practices

Managed care is also having a profound effect on the mental health delivery system. Solo practitioners lack the clinical and administrative support to treat the large numbers of severely disturbed patients who will be referred for office-based care. To earn a living, many clinicians will abandon solo practice and join multispecialty groups. Behavioral group practices will arise from the private practice community, hospital departments of psychiatry, and academic medical centers. These groups will be positioned as "carve outs" or "carve ins." In the carve out, the behavioral group practice will serve patients whose mental health care is carved out of the overall medical plan and turned over to an independent mental health provider. In the carve in, the group will be internally positioned as the department of mental health within a larger, integrated, medical delivery system.

Regardless of their relationship to the medical service provider, behavioral group practices will be similarly structured and operated. Groups will have an administrative hub that will centralize incoming referrals, manage patient information and flow, and handle the group's business matters. Clinical sites will be scattered around a wide geographic area as satellite offices. This structure is commonly referred to as a "group without walls." Each site will be responsible for routine and emergency mental health services. Specialty services will be available on referral to more centralized locations.

Groups undergo a predictable developmental process as they expand and mature. They typically begin at a single site as a coalition of independent clinicians. Growth occurs through the addition of clinicians at the original site, and later through the inclusion of clinicians practicing at geographically different locations. Over time, these informal arrangements evolve into legal, formal entities to improve efficiencies and gain access to contracts and capital.

A popular form for these arrangements is the independent practice association. In this type of association, independent clinicians often practicing at different locations unite to form a network that provides services to a specific population of patients. Membership in the independent practice association is open to all willing providers—solo office-based clinicians, members of small and large group practices, and clinicians working in community services organizations.

Recently, clinicians are creating management service organizations to provide the independent practice association with the administrative functions necessary to run the clinical delivery system and the business of the practice.

These structures give clinicians a vehicle for participating in a wide range of relationships with providers and payers. They can even transform themselves into managed care organizations and bid directly for contracts with employers and public sector patients. Already, group practices are expanding and consolidating into regional networks in search of increased market share. As this happens, the distinction between behavioral group practices, independent practice associations, management service organizations, and managed care organizations will become blurred.

Patient Access, Intake, and Triage

Regardless of the structure of the practice, patients must be able to gain access to care at any time and from any place. The telephone is the behavioral group practice's lifeline and most significant access tool. Effective intake and patient triage are crucial to the operation of behavioral group practices. Groups without walls must have a centralized access point. Intake personnel will need to be available 24 hours per day, 7 days per week, to ensure emergency intervention and hospital diversion. The intake process is both administrative and clinical. Administrative functions include verifying insurance coverage and benefits, initiating patient records, and referral of routine cases.

Crisis situations demand skillful clinical triage. As services along the continuum of care become more available and sophisticated, the triage agent will become increasingly important. Essential skills for the triage clinician include the ability to evaluate a clinical situation rapidly and to identify the point within the group practice or over the continuum of care where the patient can be best served. The triage agent must be assured immediate access to a psychiatrist. This psychiatrist can provide telephone consultation to the triage agent, face-to-face evaluation of the patient, or the prompt initiation of medication, when necessary.

Behavioral Group Practices: Characteristics

As groups of providers contract to offer care to vast numbers of "covered lives," they are discovering that providing clinical services and managing their practices are no longer synonymous. In the future, clinicians will provide care supported by managers and administrative staff. Behavioral group practices must have the following clinical characteristics to be attractive to payers and to deliver quality care:

- Twenty-four-hour, 7-days-a-week, coverage for evaluation and hospital diversion
- Full range of outpatient services for children, adolescent, and adult patients
- Staffing by multispecialty providers, including psychiatrists, psychologists, social workers, and certified addiction counselors, to ensure diversity of clinical skills and fee schedules
- Clinicians who are "willing providers" of managed behavioral care services at every level of care
- Medication management, medical/psychiatric evaluation, and other specialty services
- Familiarity with and access to a wide range of services along a continuum of care
- Access to intensive outpatient chemical dependency services, either in-house or on referral, to avoid unnecessary admissions
- Psychological testing when medically necessary
- Willingness to develop innovative programs for patients with special needs (e.g., a population with a high incidence of persistent mental illness will require different programs than one with a high incidence of substance abuse or AIDS)
- Internal utilization review and case management
- Ability to integrate outcomes data and quality assurance measurements into clinical decision making

If groups intend to take responsibility for large populations, bid for contracts, or take on financial risk, they or their management service organizations will need to have the following administrative characteristics:

- Full economic and operational integration to maximize efficiency
- Computerized management and medical information systems to provide access to the data necessary to track the clinical and financial performance of the group
- Professional management and administration to permit administrators to run the practice while clinicians provide care

- Centralized billing and collections to generate hard-copy bills for patients and insurers with the possibility of electronic transfer of data and money
- Centralized intake system to channel patients by specialty need, geographic area, and state of emergency
- State-of-the-art patient communications system with a live voice to guarantee easy access and the opportunity for triage and to ensure patient satisfaction
- Internal quality assurance programs to identify quality indicators that are routinely monitored by clinicians and administrators
- Ability to measure patient outcomes to ensure the desired outcomes
- Guidelines, policies, and procedures that support the clinical, administrative, and financial mission of the group to ensure uniformity over the entire group practice
- Access to adequate capital to support the clinical service responsibility and business interests of the group

Major Challenges

This is a time that demands flexibility on the part of mental health professionals. We are being asked, even expected, to replace the time-honored, weekly 50-minute session with varied treatment settings and sessions of varying frequency and length. Episodic treatments and group interventions offer promise for many patients. Clinicians must be willing to experiment—with attention to clinical outcomes—so that treatment guidelines are ultimately available to suggest which treatments are best for which patients and which conditions.

If 20% of patients consume 80% of the mental health resources (Patterson 1994), we should first focus attention on improving our ability to identify these high-cost, high-risk patients. Savings generated with these patients can then flow into preventive care. It may take up to 5 years for preventive interventions to show benefits, such as with families undergoing separations and divorce or families struggling with severe medical illness (Warden 1994). Because a 5-year period extends beyond most managed care contracts, preventive care is now being ignored.

Training clinicians and managers to use the continuum must be a high priority. It is especially challenging to train clinicians in short-term therapy when trainees have diminished opportunity to draw on experience with long-term treatments. Clinicians need to learn that more is not always better. At the same time, managers need to recognize when less is not preferable. Older clinicians face particular difficulty in adapting their skills and experience to time-effective treatments and a population-based perspective. Professional organizations could sponsor such retraining.

As outpatient care is shifted from the solo practitioner's office into large group practices and networks, unforeseen administrative problems will arise. An enormous volume of information, both clinical and management, must be processed. The devil is in the details—details that permit the system to operate on everyone's behalf. Stabilizing a manic patient in the office is possible only with rapid access to laboratory data. Failure to verify insurance eligibility, bill, and collect for services rendered, or to utilize and generate outcomes data, will have grave clinical and financial consequences.

In the face of diminishing resources, clinicians are struggling to develop new treatment skills and to recreate their delivery system. Meeting this challenge can make this painful era for the profession into an era of opportunity for our patients.

References

Beck AT, Rush JA, Shaw BF, et al: Cognitive Therapy of Depression. New York, Guilford, 1979

Bennett MJ: The importance of teaching the principles of managed care. Behavioral Healthcare Tomorrow 2:28–32, 1993

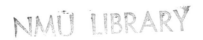

Briggs J, Peat FD: Turbulent Mirror: An Illustrated Guide to Chaos Theory and the Science of Wholeness. New York, Harper & Row, 1989

Budman SH: Treating Time Effectively (videotape and monograph). New York, Guilford, 1994

Budman SH, Armstrong E: Training for managed care settings: how to make it happen. Psychotherapy 29:416–421, 1992

Budman SH, Gurman AS: Theory and Practice of Brief Therapy. New York, Guilford, 1988

DeShazer S: Putting Differences to Work. New York, WW Norton, 1992

England MJ: From fee-for-service to accountable health plans, in Allies and Adversaries: The Impact of Managed Care on Mental Health Services. Edited by Schreter RK, Sharfstein SS, Schreter CA. Washington, DC, American Psychiatric Press, 1994, pp 3–8

Patterson DY: Outpatient services, in Allies and Adversaries: The Impact of Managed Care on Mental Health Services. Edited by Schreter RK, Sharfstein SS, Schreter CA. Washington, DC, American Psychiatric Press, 1994, pp 51–60

Warden G: Closing plenary address. Presented at the Behavioral Health Care Tomorrow Conference, Washington, DC, September 14, 1994

3 Home-Based Services

Samuel Moy, Ph.D.
H. Edmund Pigott, Ph.D.

Ms. J was a 26-year-old woman referred for hospitalization Friday morning by her employer's Employee Assistance Program (EAP) counselor due to bizarre behavior and crying episodes at work. A Positive Alternatives to Hospitalization (PATH) psychologist saw the patient at the work site within 1 hour of referral. The severely depressed patient had very low self-esteem, suicidal ideation, and panic attacks and reported having not slept for 3 nights following the breakup with her boyfriend of several years. The patient lived at home with her retired parents and had one prior psychiatric hospitalization. The psychologist

- Assessed the patient's psychiatric status and risk using PATH's Risk Assessment scale and implemented PATH's treatment protocol for suicidal patients
- Spent 2 hours actively listening to the patient to form a therapeutic alliance, elicit relevant treatment information, and develop a treatment plan for crisis stabilization
- Met with the patient and her parents at home to ensure adequate supervision over the weekend and to mobilize their participation in the treatment plan

27

- Arranged for a same-day evaluation by a PATH psychiatrist for medication and treatment plan consultation
- Provided home visits over the weekend for crisis intervention, monitored her response to medication, monitored mental status and suicide risk, ensured treatment plan compliance, and began training the patient in problem solving, relaxation, and cognitive therapy to cope with and solve her problematic symptoms and life situation
- Provided the patient 24-hour-a-day access to her PATH clinician and on-site availability to the patient and her parents
- Coordinated her return to work on a part-time basis with the employer's EAP program and her return to full-time employment shortly thereafter
- Provided problem-focused outpatient psychotherapy and medication monitoring after the patient was stabilized

Home-based services (HBS) are being "rediscovered" as a valuable treatment approach. In the continuum of behavioral health services, HBS programs are usually seen as being more intensive than traditional outpatient services but less intensive than inpatient hospitalization. These services were successfully implemented during the height of the community mental health movement in 1960s and early 1970s. HBS programs are reemerging presently as a high-quality, cost-effective treatment option for a variety of patient populations.

Although there is a wide range of services that fall within the HBS continuum, they all share several common characteristics. As the name implies, HBS are offered to patients in their homes or other settings (e.g., school, workplace). In contrast to more traditional forms of care, HBS programs emphasize outreach and working with patients in their natural environment. This provides clinicians a richer and more complete picture of their patients' problems and resources, as well as the social and physical environment in which they live. Such services reduce barriers to access and help to engage into treatment patients and their families who might otherwise avoid getting help in a more traditional setting.

Second, HBS programs are goal focused and often use an intensive crisis intervention approach to treatment. Such services are used when less intensive levels of care have been ineffective. Intensive in-home crisis intervention services seek to stabilize the patient, thereby averting the need for institution-based care. These services are focused on resolving the crisis that is precipitating the need for more intensive care. In addition to crisis intervention, there is a growing interest in using a range of HBS for services such as triage and assessment, brief therapy, and supportive treatment for various patient populations.

Third, HBS programs provide a significant amount of clinical case management services. HBS programs provide patients both behavioral health services as well as assistance in accessing necessary social services that support their recovery. This includes interventions such as patient advocacy, vocational/employment support, resource networking, and helping to provide or arrange for "concrete" services (e.g., transportation, financial management, housing).

Although HBS programs share these characteristics, they also represent a wide continuum of interventions. Such programs fall into three broad types of home-based care based on the targeted patient population, treatment goals, and type of HBS treatment. Table 3–1 summarizes these three types of HBS programs.

First, for the multiproblem chronically and persistently mentally ill patient, and/or the medically compromised mentally ill homebound patient, HBS are offered to prevent psychiatric relapse and provide some minor medical treatment. Usually these patients are served by state-funded mental health agencies or by private, community mental health centers. Current examples of HBS programs serving this patient population are assertive community treatment teams and mobile crisis units of community mental health clinics. Other frequent providers of such care are Visiting Nurse Associations. These services are provided by social workers, nurses, and home health aides. Collateral psychiatric and psychological services are readily available through traditional office-based providers working in close conjunction with the HBS program staff. Such services minimize psychiatric relapse by providing medication monitoring, clinical case management services, and intermittent crisis intervention on an ongoing basis for chronically mentally ill patients.

The second type of HBS program works with the child welfare population. The goals of these services are to avert the need for out-of-home placement due to abuse, neglect, or psychiatric problems in the child and/or parent. Such "family preservation services" are based on the belief that in most cases it is in the child's best interest to remain with his or her family rather than to be placed in a foster home or some other institutional care. These programs strive to teach parents more effective parenting skills, to reduce and stop abuse or neglect, and to create a more nurturing home environment. These programs address both the issue that precipitated the referral (e.g., child abuse) as well as working with the family to develop specific skills (e.g., commu-

Table 3–1.   Types of home-based care

Patient population	Goals of treatment	Type of treatment	Current example
Multiproblem chronically mentally ill or medically compromised mentally ill	Relapse prevention, maintenance, and/or treatment of medical condition	Community outreach and psychiatric home health	Mobile crisis teams, assertive community treatment, Visiting Nurse Association
Child welfare	Decrease abuse, neglect, and need for out-of-home placements	Family preservation, parent training, clinical and concrete services	Homebuilders
Acute psychiatric	Acute stabilization, alternative to inpatient psychiatric hospitalization	Crisis intervention	Positive Alternatives to Hospitalization

nication skills). There is often a mix of both clinical services (e.g., anger management) and "concrete" services (e.g., helping the parents arrange transportation to a medical appointment). HBS providers generally are master's- and bachelor's-level trained clinicians and behavioral home health aides. A highly successful example of one such HBS program is Homebuilders, based in Seattle, Washington. Homebuilders provides care in several counties in Washington state, and its model of family preservation services has been replicated nationally (Whittaker et al. 1988).

The third type of HBS program is designed for psychiatric patients in acute crisis. Typically, these patients have a moderately successful baseline functioning level and are not suffering from a chronic mental illness (e.g., patients tend to be employed and are covered by commercial health insurance). Such patients present with an acute crisis in their life that may require hospitalization for them to be safely stabilized. The in-home crisis intervention services are recognized as highly effective from both a clinical and cost perspective for a variety of patient populations (Pigott and Trott 1993). There is a growing body of literature supporting the clinical efficacy of such services as an alternative to psychiatric hospitalization for many patients.

PATH is an example of this third type of HBS program. PATH contracts with managed care companies to provide patients with intensive in-home crisis intervention services designed to avert the need for psychiatric hospitalization. PATH uses a multidisciplinary team approach in treating these high-risk patients. PATH providers are psychologists, social workers, nurses, and psychiatrists who have a broad range of clinical experience and expertise in crisis intervention, triage, and treatment.

Various sources refer patients to PATH's intensive crisis intervention HBS program. The key admission criterion is assessment by someone, usually another mental health provider or case manager, that the patient is in significant distress and is in need of psychiatric hospitalization for intensive treatment. Typically, referrals are made by emergency room staff who have medically cleared a patient but believe the patient needs intensive psychiatric treatment and/or hospitalization. Referrals are also initiated by the patient, family members, employer or EAP staff, school personnel, or other mental health professionals who are treating the patient. For example, the patient might be in routine outpatient psychotherapy with a mental health professional and, due to a situational crisis or acute exacerbation of a chronic condition, the patient becomes more symptomatic and suicidal. At this point, the treating clinician is actively considering hospitalization.

These patients are usually covered by managed care health plans that require preauthorization for hospital admission. The managed care organization's case manager gathers the relevant clinical data from the referral source and then refers the patient for evaluation by the intensive in-home crisis intervention treatment program before authorizing an inpatient admission.

Referrals are accepted by the PATH program 24 hours a day, 7 days a week. For emergency referrals, the patient is seen on site within 1 hour of the referral. The crisis therapist travels to wherever the patient is located. This can be the patient's home, work site, or school. Crisis therapists also see patients at the emergency room, hospital admission office, other therapist's office, or any other appropriate location. The crisis therapist makes a careful assessment of the patient and determines the appropriate level of care deemed clinically necessary for the patient. This may mean hospitalizing the patient because of an inability to treat the patient safely on an intensive in-home basis. However, in the majority of cases, patients can be effectively and safely treated on an intensive outpatient basis, thus avoiding the need for hospitalization.

Admission Criteria

The following are PATH's admission guidelines for its home-based crisis intervention program:

- Relevant provider(s) and/or referring case manager certifies that without PATH's crisis intervention service the patient's condition warrants hospitalization.
- Alternatives to PATH's crisis intervention services, including traditional, less intensive outpatient services, have been unsuccessful or inappropriate.
- Patient and family consent to PATH's services to avert or discontinue hospitalization and must be available and willing to receive PATH's services.
- Appropriate referrals include but are not limited to the following:

  - Severe conduct problems in children and adolescents
  - Suicidal problems or behaviors in children, adolescents, and adults
  - Moderate to severe disturbances in thought, mood, and/or behavior in children, adolescents, and adults

PATH reserves the right to refer elsewhere persons not meeting guidelines for admission. When the severity of the case cannot be adequately treated on an intensive outpatient basis, the patient is admitted to an inpatient facility for treatment. Patients with the following problems cannot be treated appropriately:

- Patients with an active and persistent intent to harm self or others (e.g., patients requiring one-to-one supervision on inpatient psychiatric units)
- Patients who meet legal criteria for involuntary commitment to a psychiatric hospital (e.g., imminent danger to self or others; grave disability to the extent that the patient cannot care for basic needs of living)
- Patients with severe manic, paranoid, and/or psychotic symptoms
- Patients whose reality testing is significantly impaired and/or whose behavior is severely disorganized
- PATH provider determines home-based crisis intervention services are contraindicated for patient and/or family

- Minors without an adult family member available and willing to participate in treatment
- Patients who are unable or unwilling to give informed consent for their treatment

The typical PATH referral is a patient with a history of outpatient or inpatient treatment who is facing some significant crisis in his or her life. This crisis triggers a significant increase in the patient's psychiatric symptoms. These patients usually have a major affective disorder with significant suicidal ideation. Often, there is also an underlying personality disorder or substance abuse problem. As the crisis continues and the patient's ability to cope and overall functioning worsen, the patient's symptoms become more severe. This is when the patient presents for hospitalization and is referred to PATH for evaluation and treatment.

Treatment Goals

A number of critical overarching clinical goals are pursued with patients in intensive HBS programs. First, successful crisis intervention services are built on the foundation of a solid therapeutic alliance between the patient and therapist. This clinical process goal is achieved by the therapist being trained in and successfully implementing rapid therapeutic engagement techniques. By the end of the initial visit, the patient and available family members have developed a solid therapeutic relationship with the therapist. This is achieved by spending substantial time listening to, and understanding, the presenting problems from the patient's and family's perspectives. This typically takes 2 or more hours of face-to-face contact. Although this is an obvious goal, its importance is often neglected by today's busy clinicians. Many HBS patients and their families frequently indicate they have not felt so well understood in their previous treatment. Furthermore, at the point of emotional crisis, a solid therapeutic alliance provides help, relief, and hope to the patient and family.

Developing a strong therapeutic alliance helps achieve several other important clinical goals. The time spent listening to and supporting patients and their families helps them to defuse their negative affect (e.g., anger, frustration, hopelessness). This process helps the patient and family more quickly regain their baseline emotional, cognitive, and behavioral functioning.

By actively listening, the therapist also gains a significant amount of clinical information, both subjective and objective, from the patient and family. Because the visit takes place in the patient's home and without the typical time constraints of traditional outpatient treatment, a wealth of information is more easily obtained than by interviewing the patient in an office. Although the in-home provider still needs to complete a formal assessment of the patient's mental status, suicidal risk, and overall level of functioning, much data are available during this "informal" interviewing. Additionally, by listening carefully, strategic interventions can be successfully developed and implemented because such interventions are based on working with the patient and family "where they are."

The second overarching clinical goal of HBS programs is to complete a careful assessment of the patient and family. Such patients tend to be high-risk cases requiring skillful and thorough assessment, diagnosis, and treatment planning. This is achieved by careful selection and preservice training of HBS providers. PATH's HBS providers are thoroughly trained in using its risk assessment and treatment protocols, thereby ensuring a high degree of consistency in their clinical decision making, treatment planning, and treatment services.

In the PATH program, by the end of the first visit, the risk assessment is complete, and a treatment plan has been developed in collaboration with the patient and family. The patient's and family's physical safety is of primary concern. Patient suicidal and/or homicidal risks are carefully assessed, and "no-harm" agreements are routine interventions with this population. Although averting hospitalizations is a desired goal of the PATH program, this does not inappropriately influence providers' clinical decision making. Indeed, depending on the referral source, approximately 20%–30% of cases referred to PATH's HBS program are hospitalized at intake.

The third overarching goal of HBS programs is to provide crisis intervention services as an alternative to hospitalization or other out-of-home placement, where clinically appropriate. Conceptualizing the need for hospitalization as a crisis provides a framework for effectively treating the patient and family. Crisis intervention services delivered in the home can treat a wide range of moderate to severe behavioral health and family problems. Crisis services are available to patients and families 7 days a week, 24 hours a day. Patients and families in crisis receive multiple contacts per week. These programs are designed to eliminate as many barriers to treatment as possible by providing on-site services. Therapists provide intensive, flexible, multimodal treatment to patients and families. Services are problem focused, designed to empower patients and their families to cope with problems in living.

A wide range of services is immediately available to the patient and family. These services include individual, family, and group treatment; multiple home or office visits per week; and rapid psychiatric evaluation and treatment. Such intensive services permit most crisis patients and families to be safely and effectively treated on an outpatient basis.

Well-designed and carefully implemented intensive HBS programs are extremely powerful and clinically robust. For example, PATH's experience shows that approximately 75% of patients in acute crisis can be successfully treated on an intensive, outpatient basis, with only 25% actually requiring hospitalization. Other HBS programs and studies have similar results for averting the need for hospitalization or out-of-home placement (e.g., the Homebuilders program). Providing intensive treatment in the patients' natural environment gives providers immediate feedback regarding the effectiveness of their interventions. Treatment interventions can then be modified to best meet the patients' and families' needs.

Depending on patients' specific needs, a range of in-home interventions can be used. For acutely disturbed patients, the frequency and duration of contact are high. This high frequency of contact is accomplished by multiple visits at home, in the office, and over the telephone. Patients in acute crisis are seen when needed, for as much time as is needed to stabilize them. Other less severely disturbed patients may only need a single in-home intervention and then can be quickly transitioned into routine outpatient care. Nonetheless, even for these patients, the critical intervention occurs during the intake visit. At the point of crisis, patients and families are often much more amenable to change when approached in an effective and respectful manner. By providing convenient, easily accessed, and intensive services, most patients in acute crisis are significantly helped.

A key treatment strategy of HBS is to involve the patient's social support systems (i.e., family, significant others, friends) in treatment whenever possible. The patient's social support systems are recruited, supported, and empowered to help the patient resolve the crisis rather than these social supports being supplanted by hospitalization. For example, when appropriate and necessary, the PATH program teaches willing family members to provide an "in-home holding bed" for the patient. This essentially provides a highly structured and supportive home situation to help the patient to de-escalate safely. When this is done, the therapist remains in very close contact with the patient and family.

Most HBS programs also work to maintain the continuity of patient care. Thus, although a patient and family may see a number of different professionals (e.g., psychiatrist, psychologist, group therapist), there is always one person who performs a "clinical case manager" role. This professional coordinates the patient's care and is the patient's primary therapist. This ensures a seamless service to patients and families and helps to maintain a sense of continuity in their treatment. After the patient is stabilized by the in-home crisis intervention services, the patient is referred for more routine ongoing outpatient services as needed. This provides for more effective and efficient care for the patient.

A fourth and final overarching goal of many HBS programs is to monitor and improve the quality of patient care. This is usually accomplished by obtaining pretreatment and posttreatment measures of patient functioning and collecting patient satisfaction data. At the PATH HBS program, all cases are reviewed concurrently to ensure quality of care, and case consultation and supervision occur at least weekly. Clinicians are strongly encouraged to consult colleagues whenever necessary. A senior psychologist and psychiatrist are always available for consultation to the HBS staff. Assessment and treatment protocols have been developed based on review of the available empirical and clinical literature, and clinicians are carefully trained in their use. These protocols are regularly reviewed and revised to ensure continuous quality improvement.

Outcomes Research

In a 2-year outcome analysis of PATH's HBS program, involving more than 600 health maintenance organization (HMO) patients presenting for hospitalization, Pigott and Trott (1993) found the following:

- PATH's in-home crisis intervention service averted the need for hospitalization for 81% of referred patients.
- Patients treated by PATH had a 400% lower psychiatric rehospitalization rate compared with patients not treated by PATH.
- The HMO saved an average of 18 days of hospital-based care per PATH referral.

Due to PATH's intensive crisis intervention service, the HMO experienced a 50% decrease in psychiatric inpatient days. In this era of concern for high-quality, cost-efficient care, PATH has shown that intensive HBS programs are a positive alternative to hospitalization for many acute psychiatric patients.

Critical Components to Success

Although there are many factors that contribute to the success of HBS, four are especially noteworthy. These programs are built on a set of dominant values that are important to understand and appreciate. First, these programs seek to treat patients in the least restrictive environment. This is consistent with ethical and public policy concerns. Hospitalization is both stigmatizing and fosters dependency for many patients. HBS avoid these problems by providing treatment that is physically "close" to the patient and avoids the inevitable disruption of hospitalization. Furthermore, home-based care is aimed at empowering patients and families to help themselves rather than depending on outside professionals or institutions to solve their problems. Although services are provided in the least restrictive environment, this does not mean that patients do not receive necessary and sufficient levels of care. Intensive in-home treatment often provides more direct contact between patients and providers than patients might receive on some inpatient units.

A second important value is providing care that is easy to access and readily available. HBS programs are not limited to regular "business hours." Instead, these services seek to eliminate barriers to treatment by providing on-site care, with availability 7 days a week, 24 hours a day. Too often, professional services have been designed to be convenient for the practitioner rather than the patient. Although this is less of an issue for high-functioning patients, for patients in crisis such limited access often compounds their difficulties. Easily accessible services help patients feel more confident and safe knowing that intensive help is always just a telephone call away.

A third value is using a flexible, multimodal treatment approach. Successful intensive HBS programs use a biopsychosocial treatment model. Such programs view mental health crises as precipitated by a complex interaction between personal and environmental factors, often in persons who have a genetic predisposition toward developing serious psychiatric problems. By using a flexible, multidisciplinary team approach, the patient and family are provided care that addresses the biological, psychological, and social factors involved.

Therapist flexibility is also important in this regard. Successful HBS therapists are a special group. They need to be bright, energetic, personable, and able to function under a great deal of stress. Providing care in a patient's home rather than an office can be very challenging and disorienting for the therapist. The usual boundaries of traditional mental health treatment services are absent (e.g., no therapy office when the HBS therapist is at a patient's home). This requires the therapist to be more flexible and yet remain goal focused to help the patient and family successfully resolve the problems that precipitated the crisis. While using assessment and treatment protocols, therapists still operate with a great deal of autonomy. They need to respond to patients in crisis whenever needed and thus must maintain a high degree of both professional and personal flexibility. Careful therapist selection, thorough preservice training, and extensive on-going supervision are critical factors to maintaining a successful HBS program.

A fourth value is the importance of the patient's social supports. When a patient's social supports are willing to cooperate with treatment, the patient is much more likely to have a positive outcome. Mobilizing the patient's social supports is an early treatment goal. Social supports help to reduce patient isolation, maximize treatment effects, and reduce suicide risk. Furthermore, because a patient's crises are often precipitated by interpersonal conflicts between the patient and his or her family, working with the patient's family will reduce the stress level for the patient and family alike. By actively incorporating and strengthening social supports, such high-risk patients are more likely to be safely and competently cared for on an intensive outpatient basis.

Conclusion

HBS programs are a viable, cost-effective treatment modality for many psychiatric and child welfare populations. Both public and private providers of such care recognize the clinical utility and robustness of this range of interventions. Providing successful in-home care requires careful program design and implementation. The underlying values of such programs are an important foundation for providing clinicians with the philosophical orientation and clinical perspectives to ensure program success. Well-designed alternatives to hospitalization provide high-quality and cost-effective care for many patients who in previous times would have been hospitalized. Intensive HBS programs effectively treat the majority of patients experiencing an acute psychiatric crisis while avoiding the potential iatrogenic effects of hospitalization or out-of-home placement.

Home-based treatments represent a significant change in how the mental health industry operates. This positive change is stimulated by public and private payers' desire to provide more cost-effective and high-quality treatment options for psychiatric patients and their families.

References

Pigott HE, Trott LT: Curbing behavioral health costs while enhancing the quality of patient care: the implementation of a crisis intervention, triage and treatment service in the private sector. Am J Med Qual 8:138–144, 1993

Whittaker JK, Kinney J, Tracy EM, et al (eds): Improving Practice Technology for Work With High Risk Families: Lessons From the "Homebuilders" Social Work Education Project. Seattle, WA, Center for Social Welfare Research, University of Washington, 1988

Additional Readings

Kagan R, Scholosberg S: Families in Perpetual Crisis. New York, WW Norton, 1989

Kiesler C, Sibulkin AE: Mental Hospitalization: Myths and Facts About a National Crisis. Beverly Hills, CA, Sage, 1987

4 Emergency Crisis Services

David Fassler, M.D.
Gail Hanson-Mayer, R.N., C.S., M.P.H.
Terri Hubbard, M.S., L.M.H.C.

∎ CASE 1

Mr. A receives a call at work. The call is from his 11-year-old son who is crying and stating that he just returned home from school and found his mother (Mr. A's ex-wife) asleep on the couch; the boy has been unable to wake her. He describes an empty pill bottle on the floor next to his mother. The father then calls an ambulance, which transports both the patient and the boy to the nearest hospital emergency room.

Assessment. Following medical clearance, the emergency room physician requests a psychiatric consult. A psychiatric nurse clinician then interviews the patient, speaks with her son and ex-husband, and then consults with the patient's primary care physician and therapist, as well as with the consulting psychiatrist. After completion of the assessment, the nurse then obtains approval from the managed care company for the clinically appropriate level of care.

43

Formulation. Based on information obtained from the assessment, the following were determined:

- The overdose was a suicidal gesture.
- The patient has mild suicide risk factors associated with continued vague ideation and an acute stressor.
- An inadequate support system is in place.
- The patient exhibits positive motivation to receive help.

Disposition. Placement for one night in an open respite program will allow for continued observation and crisis intervention to assist with the development of a plan that effectively deals with the stressor, increases her support system, and helps her to commit to a "safety plan." Based on the disposition, the crisis clinician, managed care company, and patient agree on the following plan:

- Discharge from respite within 24 hours
- A therapy appointment within 24–48 hours
- A concrete safety plan during crisis periods that incorporates the patient's new therapist, additional supports, and emergency services

▌ CASE 2

A school counselor contacts the local emergency services. She describes an 8-year-old female who bit another student, kicked a teacher, and attempted to isolate herself in a nearby closet. The counselor reports that the child's teachers have recently noted an increase in aggressive outbursts, including verbal threats to other children. To avoid unnecessary transport of the child, who is currently in behavioral control, the crisis clinician and school agree to a mobile evaluation.

Assessment. The clinician obtains approval from the managed care company to provide the mobile evaluation. The clinician then evaluates the child at the school, locates the mother, and obtains background information and pertinent clinical data. Following the interview with the child and her mother, the clinician consults with school personnel.

Formulation. The recent onset of the child's escalation of aggressive outbursts coincides with the mother's reunification with the child's biological father. The tumultuous history between the mother and father appears to be the most immediate stressor for the child.

Disposition. The mother agrees to family-/home-based intervention, which will be intensive and short term. Weekly outpatient treatment will be subsequently arranged for the child.

▌ CASE 3

Mr. W, a 22-year-old, arrives on site at a local emergency room; he was referred by his insurance provider. The patient states he has a problem with cocaine and cannot return to work until he receives help. He also states that he no longer has a place to live because his girlfriend evicted him from the apartment this morning. A psychiatric consultation is requested by the emergency room physician.

Assessment. The consulting psychiatric clinician evaluates the patient, obtains a full substance abuse history, and then speaks with the patient's girlfriend.

Formulation. Mr. W's recent history is marked with a number of uncompleted detoxifications secondary to against-medical-advice status. His motivation to be drug free has been assessed to be minimal, driven primarily by the girlfriend's eviction and the possible loss of his job. There is no suicidality.

Disposition. The clinician recommends attendance for 1 week at a substance abuse day treatment program, to be followed by weekly outpatient substance abuse counseling, and daily Alcoholics Anonymous/Cocaine Anonymous meetings. The managed care company agrees with the plan, concurring that an inpatient setting is not warranted.

These case studies represent a variety of situations that psychiatric emergency service personnel typically encounter.

Whether in an emergency room of a general hospital, a free-standing psychiatric emergency service, or a community setting, the goals of each provider are the same: accurate clinical assessment and the provision of cost-effective treatment.

In this chapter, we focus on the role of an emergency service within the managed care continuum. Comparisons are drawn between facility- and nonfacility-based programs, specifically with reference to both the advantages and disadvantages for managed care organizations, consumers, and emergency service programs. Finally, we address the components of a crisis program, inclusive of cost analysis and the application of quality improvement measures.

Role of Emergency Service Programs in the Managed Care System

Before managed care, emergency service programs usually provided brief intervention and assessment, relying heavily on inpatient facilities to stabilize patients. This trend appears to have been perpetuated by the virtual nonexistence of alternatives, as well as by the philosophy at the time that the highest-quality treatment was within an inpatient setting.

The health care system has undergone a radical transformation within the past 10 years. Health care providers across all continuums are now striving to keep abreast of, or ahead of, managed care. A major part of this transformation has been the continued development of innovative treatment programs for mental health and substance abuse patients. It is estimated that about 4% of insurance dollars are spent on mental health and substance abuse treatment today, as compared with a historical 10% (Pomerantz 1995). Quality cost-effective alternatives to traditional forms of treatment are paramount.

Emergency service programs for mental health and substance abuse have expanded their roles significantly in response to the need for managing a patient's care in the least intensive and the least costly fashion. To provide clinically responsible treatment options for patients, these programs must now be integrated within a continuum of services, with both affiliated and nonaffiliated programs.

Managed care has revitalized emergency service programs. It has been perhaps the sole factor that has positioned emergency services as a priority program within most mental health care provider organizations. If the emergency service program does not understand and cannot apply the principles of managed care, it will not survive and neither will its affiliated programs (i.e., inpatient, outpatient, respite).

Deinstitutionalization and a greater emphasis on short-term treatment have led to increased utilization of emergency service programs. Often a patient's entrance into the mental health system occurs after the patient has received a "crisis assessment" from an emergency service. The assessment request may result from the patient presenting him- or herself with an emergency need or from the patient's managed care company. The focus of both the crisis team and the managed care company includes the following:

● Proactivity and responsiveness to patients
● Provision of an extensive and encompassing intervention that establishes the immediate and short-term appropriate level of care
● Cooperation with a full network of quality resources

Optimal individualized care can be provided to patients, given the flexibility and creativity of both systems

Facility-Based Versus Freestanding Emergency Service Programs

Although many general hospital emergency rooms utilize their own in-house staff to provide crisis evaluations, an increasing number now contract with psychiatric consultation services. Advantages of utilizing a consultation service range from financial savings gained from reduced overhead to improved employee relations by not pulling possibly unqualified staff from their primary clinical responsibilities. Additionally, the hospital becomes known as an access site to a full continuum of mental health care, thus increasing its utilization and managed care payer mix.

Consultation programs providing mental health and substance abuse crisis services are typically managed by health care companies specializing in this area. Health care organizations that have well-developed and vertically integrated programs are positioned to secure and maintain numerous managed care contracts for the provision of crisis services.

A mental health organization that positions its crisis service within a community setting, such as a general hospital emergency department, avoids being viewed as self-serving and eliminates the perceived temptation to admit a patient to "the inpatient unit down the hall" following evaluation. This does not mean, of course, that a crisis service has no investment in referring to programs within its own network. A responsible crisis service will place importance on having a full knowledge of the organization's network of services and will then match the patient's clinical needs and level of care to a specific program. There are always patients who present with special needs or circumstances that a health care network does not provide. To meet the patient's clinical needs, the crisis service must then have a working knowledge of numerous referral programs in the community. Increasingly, referrals are primarily determined by the managed care company, which has a prearranged capitation or utilization contract with that referent. To serve as the patient's advocate, it is crucial that clinicians working for a crisis service understand managed care networks, their requirements, and their affiliated programs. Level of care criteria and program affiliations should be obtained from the various managed care companies for purposes of training crisis clinicians. Although there are subtle differences in level of care criteria among managed care companies, the commitment to quality care is the same. Each individual crisis program needs to incorporate similar levels of care criteria as policy within its own service.

Patients benefit from crisis service programs sited in community settings. There is less "stigma-factor" for those patients who are uncomfortable seeking an evaluation from a mental health agency. Additionally, patients who would have never asked for help may be identified as having a psychiatric or substance abuse problem and referred for an evaluation.

In contrast, as discussed, crisis teams that are located in the same site as their "sister programs" (e.g., inpatient, respite, observation beds, partial hospitalization) have several disadvantages. Managed care companies and patients may view crisis teams as only a mechanism to increase their own facility's census and may believe that the facility is ignoring cost-effectiveness and less intensive treatment options. However, if the crisis service is performing effectively, this perception can be changed. Crisis clinicians who accurately design treatment plans that match a patient's level of care, regardless of whether the appropriate care is within the facility's network, demonstrate this effectiveness. Referrals that include self-help groups and the patient's own support system should be regularly utilized by crisis clinicians. An organization whose crisis team is located "on site" is advantageous for the patient who requires a more intensive level of care following evaluation. Additionally, the on-site team is advantageous for the organization as it may benefit from increased economies of staff and exposure of its services.

Service Elements

Hours of Operation and Staffing

An emergency service program must operate continuously at 100% efficiency 24 hours a day. This is challenging and stressful even for seasoned staff and administrators. Education level and previous crisis experience should be strong considerations when hiring staff. Other key qualifications include a demonstrated ability to make diagnoses and formulations quickly and accurately, a wide knowledge base in mental health and substance abuse, and excellent judgment, stress tolerance, and professionalism. Additionally, hiring and training surplus staff and rotating them into the schedule will address the need for qualified clinicians to fill unexpected and sudden staffing gaps.

Mobility

Mobility to sites outside of the primary service area is tantamount to running an effective emergency service. Clinicians must be flexible when circumstances warrant mobile evaluations (e.g., jails, inpatient medical units, schools, homes). It is advantageous for crisis services to work closely with a home- and family-based crisis program that specifically provides mobile evaluations to children and their family network.

Components of the Crisis Evaluation

The crisis evaluation itself includes accurate triage, mental status examination, psychosocial history, substance abuse profile, and determination of dangerousness. During this process of information gathering and assessment, the clinician begins formulating the patient's clinical needs. After consulting with the appropriate staff on the crisis team (e.g., staff psychiatrist, supervisor), a disposition is arranged. During this process, the quality of the skills of the crisis team directly impacts the patient. The ability to assess the patient's *immediate and short-term needs* accurately will influence the level of the patient's satisfaction, commitment to treatment, and success of treatment. A crisis clinician must advocate for the patient to ensure that he or she receives the appropriate level and degree of care. It can be frustrating for patients to understand the managed care system and the treatment options now available to them. A crisis worker's role includes not only referring the patient to the appropriate program, but also educating the patient on the benefits and array of mental health and substance abuse services that exist today.

Risk Management

Emergency services is an area of high-risk management. Medical-legal documentation training should be provided on hire, and retraining should occur on a regular basis. Written evaluations are often requested by managed care companies and the agencies/hospitals accepting the patient for referral. Correspondingly, the written evaluation becomes a permanent part of the patient's medical record. It is therefore crucial that evaluations are consistent and follow a format that meets the requirements of the host facility and licensing agencies.

Cost Analysis and Staffing

The cost for operating an emergency service is variable. Location, economies of staff, agency and licensing requirements, and size all influence the financial viability of the service.

Staffing

Hiring both on-site and on-call staff is the most cost-effective way to staff emergency service programs that service approximately 100–150 patients each month. It is preferable that on-site staff work during the peak hours (mid-afternoon through late evening hours), with on-call staff covering the remaining hours. Pay scales for licensed master's-level clinicians vary across states. However, it is advisable to pay $5–$10 per hour above the standard rate for on-site time worked by on-call staff. This financial incentive is effective in recruiting and retaining on-call staff, the most difficult pool of staff to maintain. However, paying *too high* a rate for the *on-call hours* can be incentive for the clinician to request large segments of time to be on-call and then attempt to limit the actual on-site hours. Usually these staff will remain on the team for only a short time.

Administrative/Clinical Leadership

The director should preferably be a clinician with a strong clinical background and superior management and supervisory skills. The psychiatry staff should be experienced in providing crisis assessment backup. To defer the cost of maintaining a psychiatry staff, a pool of psychiatrists within an already existing system may be utilized to provide the on-site intervention.

A freestanding emergency service program will present additional financial challenges. Incorporating existing staff from other already established programs is cost-effective and ensures quality care and experienced staff.

Financial Viability

Revenue for emergency service programs may come from contracted arrangements with host sites and/or direct reimbursement by managed care companies. In either case, a reimbursement rate structure must be established that anticipates the operating costs and break-even volume of the service. Closely monitoring the financial status of the service is essential given the limited profit margin. However, when considering the financial viability of the service, the revenue generated by referrals to other services within the network must be considered.

Table 4–1 details a basic financial statement that outlines the cost associated with operating a freestanding emergency service program within a host general hospital; the program is owned and managed by a mental health organization.

Quality Improvement

Quality crisis services need to be built on a solid foundation that consists of two essential components: stabilization of the crisis and successful referral to the next appropriate level of care.

Measuring the quality of a psychiatric emergency services program can be daunting. All facets of evaluation and treatment, including structure, process, outcome, and patient variables, must be assessed to get a true picture of the quality of care delivered. Because it is overambitious to attempt such a task simultaneously, the goal should be to look at a number of criteria in each category over time (Sateia et al. 1990).

Criteria related to structural elements that are measurable for emergency service programs may include level of support available to clinicians, sufficient staffing to allow for adequate time to perform an evaluation, and work satisfaction (Sateia et al. 1990).

Criteria related to process elements include items such as assessment of diagnosis, risk, and socioeconomic class. Clinician performance is also important, although difficult, to monitor. A chart audit method is probably most widely used and is least costly; however, the content validity is low. Giving feedback to

Table 4–1. Financial statement

Operating costs:	
Program director .5FTE (inclusive of 14.96% fringe)	$28,658
On-call M.D. ($50/day × 365)	$18,250
Expenses (travel, marketing, supplies)	$1,200
On-call clinicians ($3/hr × 168 hrs/week × 52 weeks)	$26,208
On-site clinicians (50 cases/month × 2.5 hrs/case × $22/hr × 12 months)	$33,000
Total expenses	$107,316
Revenue:	
75 cases/month × $225/case × 12 months	$202,500
Net revenue (gross at 60%)	$121,500
Financial statement:	
Net revenue	$121,500
Total operating expenses	$107,316
Contribution margin	$14,184

Note. FTE = full-time equivalent.

the team as a whole and individually is effective in establishing positive changes in the performance of clinicians. Performance criteria to be assessed in psychiatric emergency cases should include identification of the primary problems and other complicating factors, an adequate medical evaluation when necessary, dangerousness/risk assessment, and an appropriate specific disposition.

Criteria related to outcome are most accurate when combined with some form of process criteria measure. Approaches most frequently employed here are measures of patient compliance with referrals and patient satisfaction surveys. Patient variables are also important to measure, as they give more meaning to structure, process, and outcome measures (Sateia et al. 1990).

A quality emergency service will collectively meet the goals of its standards of care, as well as the managed care company's goals. Clinicians demonstrating quality skills, stewardship, and advocacy for patients promote responsible patient care and satisfaction.

In summary, emergency service programs have an increasingly important role in the community, both in the private and public sector. As professionals providing crisis services, our first responsibility is to provide quality care for our patients. Orchestrating the care and treatment of patients, thereby successfully moving them from the point of crisis to the point of healing, is our goal—managing care.

References

Pomerantz JM: A managed care ethical credo: for clinicians only? Psychiatr Serv 46:329–330, 1995
Sateia M, Gustafson D, Johnson S: Quality assurance for psychiatric emergencies. Psychiatr Clin North Am 13:35–48, 1990

Additional Readings

Cooper S, Lentner T (eds): Innovations in Community Mental Health. Sarasota, FL, Professional Resource Press, 1992

Greenstone J, Yeviton S: Elements of Crisis Intervention: Crises and How to Respond to Them. New York, Van Nostrand Reinhold, 1993

Johnson K: School Crisis Management: Hands-On Guide to Training Crisis Response Teams. Alameda, CA, Hunter House, 1993

5 Community Residential Care for Adults

Richard D. Budson, M.D.

As he sat in the waiting area, even though he was delusional and paranoid, Thomas, a 20-year-old stock boy in a local supermarket, was aware enough to be frightened by his immediate reality. He had been to this hospital admitting office once before—about 2 years ago. The immediate consequence was an incarceration in an inpatient unit from which he was unable to leave for 4 months. Having had tardive dyskinesia, and unable to take any of the existing antipsychotic medications, his symptoms were difficult to control. He watched as a stream of other patients came and went as he continued to be locked up. Back at his home, his father was a disabled veteran, bedridden and helpless. His mother, working nights as an office cleaner, was always exhausted and unable to cope with her son's psychotic episodes. Living in isolation, Thomas had no friends to speak of and was deficient in social skills. This visit to the hospital turned out to be different. During an overnight stay in the triage unit, he was given a new drug, clozapine, and his symptoms rapidly improved. The next day, instead of being sent to a hospital inpatient unit, he was sent to a residence—Hopeful House—abutting the hospital grounds. It felt like a warm home, with helpful, kind staff and a relatively stable group of fellow residents who were able to share feelings with Thomas as he more quickly regained his preexisting health. After only 3 weeks in the residence, Thomas was back at work at the supermarket; he continued to live in the residence another month, learning how to care and share with his housemates. Then, instead of moving back home, he moved into a cooperative apartment with three other residents who were his first real friends in 8 years, since his first psychotic episode. He and his friends looked after each other, and Thomas had never felt better.

This vignette illustrates a chronic relapsing serious psychotic disorder in a patient with inadequate family and social supports, with resulting deficient social skills. Instead of being treated with traditional hospitalization and returned to a home devoid of opportunities for growth, the patient is rehabilitated in two different levels of residential care, resulting in true life change. This illustrates the therapeutic power of the modern hospital as a system of care.

Redefining the Psychiatric Hospital as a System of Care

The modern psychiatric hospital can no longer be conceptualized as a "hospital" alone. Rather, it should be considered a "system of care" with an array of alternatives that ensure the patient receives the least restrictive treatment necessary. An additional attribute of this is also likely to be the lowest-cost service necessary to care for patients properly. This helps patients and families because it conserves their mental health benefits, which are dearly needed over time when they are confronted with an illness that by its nature is a chronic relapsing condition.

Accomplishing the combined goals of least restrictive and lowest-cost alternatives creates another new concept for psychiatric hospitals. The goal is no longer to "admit" a patient to the inpatient service of the hospital; rather, it is to "triage" the patient into the minimal service requirement necessary to restore health. Included in these services is an array of residential care alternatives.

Selecting the Least Restrictive Setting for the New Patient

Even if hospitalization is deemed to be required, the first issue is to shorten its duration. This can be accomplished by changing the traditional goals of psychiatric hospitalization. From a goal of in-depth personality change, the hospital can move toward rapid crisis intervention into the sociobiological system that precipitated the episode, firm establishment of the diagnosis, proper implementation of pharmacological treatment, stabilization, and early discharge.

However, it has become apparent to providers of inpatient care that certain patients are at high risk for longer hospital stays through a combination of factors. These include 1) unusual acuity of the initial illness; 2) chronicity of a severe illness previously manifest, often identifiable through previous readmissions to a psychiatric hospital; and 3) extremely poor community supports, including acutely dysfunctional families. Because this high-risk group presents both a potential clinical problem and a special economic problem for the private psychiatric hospital, patients in these categories should be considered for community residential care at the outset of clinical evaluation. Clinically, the capacity to render effective care in noninpatient settings for these difficult patients prevents unnecessary long-term hospitalization with the adverse clinical consequences of desocialization, stigmatization, and unnecessary removal from more normalized settings. Economically, the lack of nonhospital treatment alternatives would threaten the hospital's ability to go "at risk" in both its health maintenance organization capacity and in its low "per-episode cost" contracts. It is clear that if a significantly lower-cost alternative to hospitalization were available to those potential patient "outliers" who could not be discharged home, then the hospital system would have a chance of fiscal viability (Budson 1994).

The new system of care, then, would create a low-cost system of care and treatment that still permitted longer-term psychiatric rehabilitation for the most seriously disabled patients in greatest need. The components of the system would include 1) significant shortening of average length of hospitalization with redefined goals; 2) an array of community residential care facilities for different specialized populations and with varying levels of acuity; 3) partial hospitalization, often operating in close conjunction with residential alternatives; and 4) ambulatory/outpatient care services that sustain patient stability, preventing recidivism through relapse prevention measures.

A New Role for Community Residential Care

This reconstellation of the entire care system calls on community residential care to play an entirely new role from that which it was conceptualized to play when it emerged as an innovative health care component 25 years ago (Budson 1973, 1978, 1979; Glasscote et al. 1971; Landy and Greenblatt 1965; Raush and Raush 1968). In the era of the late 1960s and 1970s, long-term hospitalization was the rule rather than the exception. The psychiatric community residence was used almost exclusively as an aftercare setting following hospitalization. It offered "normalization," a real-life experience in a supportive family-like setting located truly within the community. Average lengths of stay in the community residence were 6 or 7 months, during which the residents learned social living skills that allowed them to move out in clusters into shared apartments and other types of community living (Budson 1978). The community residence was characterized as creating an "extended psychosocial kinship system" (Budson and Jolley 1978) that spun off clusters of ex-residents who sustained health and prevented recidivism through continued relatedness in their postcommunity residence experience. The staffing of the community residence was almost universally a live-in staff that slept overnight. Patients with psychotic disorders had illnesses that generally were under good control, or the patients would still be in the hospital.

Instead of this unidimensional use of the halfway house as an aftercare facility, we have today an array of residential alternatives. These include the high-intensity community residence, the long-term group residence, the high-expectation halfway house, and the cooperative apartment. Patients may enter these programs directly from the community, after a brief evaluation in the hospital triage facility, after a 24- to 48-hour inpatient stabilization, or after a 10- to 20-day hospitalization.

Community residential facilities thus may represent a continuum themselves, within an overall continuum serving different patient populations, differentiated both by diagnosis and by level of disability, with a range of costs depending primarily on staffing intensity (Budson 1990, 1994). There may be specialized programs developed for special patient groups: for persons recovering from substance abuse, for adolescents, for women, and for affective and character disorders. The largest group of patients needing community residential care, however, is the group with severe psychotic disorders. The system of care includes a short-term inpatient unit, which discharges patients within 10 days to a high-intensity community residential treatment facility, which in turn can step patients down into another slightly lower-intensity long-term community residence, which can discharge patients into a community-based halfway house. Finally, we have cooperative apartments with only visiting staff. No one patient need go through the entire array; rather, patients are selected for entry to a facility according to functional level and discharged to that setting for which they are ready.

Close integration of the inpatient care with the acute-care residence and affiliated partial hospital is helpful. This rapid movement of patients has impacted the professional satisfaction and training of mental health professionals. When patients are hospitalized for only a week or two, neither the staff nor trainees, if only on the inpatient unit, have an opportunity to witness the course of illness through ultimate reintegration of the psyche and instrumental life improvement. By being able to follow patients clinically into the residential care system, trainees will have an opportunity to learn the evolution of the disease course.

Some Issues and Principles Unique to Residential Care

When one is building a residential program within the context of a traditional psychiatric hospital, a great deal of energy and thought needs to be applied to create the most therapeutic clinical milieu in the most efficient manner. This is not always easy. Forces to maintain the status quo and to include established staffing and professional patterns can be quite intense. In general, there is only one to one-and-a-half full-time equivalent nurses for a 20-bed high-intensity program. Mental health counselors, who are well-trained college graduates with degrees in psychology, are utilized in clusters of two to three under the supervision of psychologists or social workers working as a team with six to eight severely disturbed patients. This system maximizes care with the minimum of cost. Second, a case manager system is in place whereby the professional supervising the counselors leads the team and oversees the direction of the care. This system removes redundancy or duplication of effort that occurs in less organized systems. Third, I have found the most effective model to be transdisciplinary, whereby all of the various mental health professionals, psychiatrists, psychologists, social workers, rehabilitation counselors, and nurses are case managers, with their special expertise utilized only when needed. This transdisciplinary model is distinct from the hospital model, where the psychologist does testing, the social worker sees the family, the rehabilitation counselor only tests for vocational readiness, and so on.

It should also be noted that there is a whole sequence of administrative issues that differentiate community residential care from hospital care. The following elements are unique to community residential care facilities: licensing, Joint Commission on Accreditation of Healthcare Organizations accreditation, building codes, zoning, nursing medication regulations, quality assurance, staffing/job descriptions, finances/rates/budgets, medical records, and marketing.

Of particular clinical significance is the fact that residential care facilities are open units. There are no locked doors. Patients, therefore, must be safe enough from harming themselves or others to handle an open unit. Furthermore, they cannot be so psychotic as to be confused and in danger of wandering off disoriented.

The typical locations and structures of these facilities vary. The high-intensity community residence is best located within the hospital campus so that all of the emergency health care backups are readily available to support patients being treated in an open setting. Sometimes this facility is placed in a space that was formerly an inpatient setting, reconfigured into a residence largely with the use of more homelike furnishings. The long-term community residence is best developed in an old, large house. It is suitably placed either in the community or on the grounds of a hospital, if there are such "cottages" available, as are at some older psychiatric hospitals. High-expectation halfway houses and cooperative apartments are essentially in existing dwellings in the community.

Different Types of Community Residences

The most recently developed high-intensity community residence is designed from the outset to take patients who have had either no hospitalization whatsoever or a brief admission of no more than 2 weeks. It requires staff who are experienced in treating very ill psychiatric patients, who have good clinical judgment, and who can make many decisions expeditiously with confidence.

Three important clinical tasks are accomplished during the hospitalization of a patient with an acute psychotic episode. First, the patient is carefully medically cleared; for example, any underlying organic illness that may or may not have psychiatric components is identified and treated as necessary. Second, the patient's psychiatric symptoms are moderately brought under control clinically; for example, the patient is no longer violent either to him- or herself or others or is no longer destructive to property and is coherent enough to reason with. Third, an appropriate psychopharmacological regimen is established.

While hospitalization continues, the acute intensive-care residence uniquely requires that a clinician on its team be involved with the inpatient team from the time of admission so that key elements are known at the time of referral to the residence: the precipitant of the episode; the nature of the successful interpersonal, milieu, and pharmacological interventions; the rationale of the psychopharmacological regimen; the status of the family's involvement, support, and capacity to receive the patient back home; and the likely further sites for ultimate disposition of the patient.

With these tasks accomplished, the acute community residence can take the patient. The residence itself is unique in its more intensive staffing than other residences. There is around-the-clock awake staff experienced in and ready to deal with patients who have not yet fully recovered from acute psychotic disorders and who have been only recently pharmacologically stabilized. Nurses in this high-intensity facility are available around the clock to assist in adjusting the newly started medication regimens or in monitoring for side effects. Community meetings occur daily instead of weekly. For some patients, life skills acquisition is the first priority of the program. For others, rehabilitation counseling and occupational therapy are a major emphasis, as vocational readiness is a programmatic priority. Instead of a 6-month average stay in the residence, some patients are certified by the third-party payer managed care arm for only 30 days of care, with renewal based on concurrent weekly or biweekly intervals. A multidisciplinary team of professionals supports and supervises the staff of counselors. Affiliated partial hospitalization programs engage the patient in an intense daily program of group rehabilitation meetings. The goal of this program is to allow for stabilization of the antipsychotic treatment plan developed in the inpatient program immediately before transfer. By 30 days, the most prominent psychotic symptoms of the patient are characteristically abated, and the patient is therefore ready for discharge to home. Alternatively, if the home setting is not adequately supportive or stable, or if a family is intolerant of the family member with a recurrent psychotic disorder who returns home, then referral to a less intense community residence is made, possibly to the long-term community residence for acquisition of needed life skills to permit more independent living. The entire milieu works with purpose and intensity to facilitate a rapid recompensation to a previous premorbid state.

The long-term group residence provides care that is in the mode of more traditional community residential care. It is usually used for those patients who are among the most severely and chronically impaired. It may act as a "step-down" facility for patients leaving the high-intensity residence after 30 days. Alternatively, these may be ambulatory schizophrenic patients who often have not had beneficial therapeutic results, despite a wide variety of pharmacological and psychotherapeutic efforts. Around-the-clock supervision and programming are required for these patients. The staffing in this type of program is usually around-the-clock shifts of counselors, usually two at a time on duty, with a single awake person on duty through the sleeping hours at night. A multidisciplinary professional staff complement during the day facilitates the various rehabilitative components required in the program. Thus, included are a psychiatrist, psychiatric nurse, social worker, rehabilitation counselor, and psychologist.

Program components provided in the group residence include life skills as well as prevocational skills training. These skills include all of those involved in daily living, such as dressing appropriately, maintaining personal hygiene, and managing money, and those skills needed in the community, such as using transportation, shopping, banking, and utilizing community resources, including sheltered workshops, libraries, community centers, and recreation and entertainment.

It is in the long-term group residence that some of the clinical attributes traditionally unique to community residential care are seen. Relapse prevention is one of the cornerstones of this facility. The long-term stay allows observation and documentation of characteristic pathological behavioral patterns in a particular patient that presage exacerbation of his or her psychotic symptoms. These patterns are subject to unusually early therapeutic intervention because they occur under the direct observation of trained staff. Furthermore, it should be noted that in carefully evaluating the patient, the early signs of impending decompensation unique to that patient are also elicited so that the staff is alert to the eventuality of their appearance. Examples of this would include a patient who characteristically does not smoke suddenly begins to smoke cigarettes incessantly or a patient who had been meticulous, neat, and punctual becomes messy and misses or is late for his or her obligations.

Clinicians with experience in this type of care believe that these subtle changes would most likely either be missed if the patient were seen only in outpatient visits or would be discovered so late in the course of decompensation that hospitalization could not be prevented. Therefore, the rectifying intervention can be made earlier than would otherwise be possible. Intervening earlier also is beneficial because the patient has not yet become so psychotic as to prevent him or her from becoming a true collaborator in the endeavor of relapse prevention. This, then, is a new learning experience for the patient, who can, in this unique setting, be engaged in the process of learning how to take care of his or her own illness—especially when decompensation is impending. In this context, the patient gains mastery of the primitive parts of the psyche. All of this represents a powerful therapeutic event that could not have occurred in other settings.

In addition to being alert to the early signs of relapse, the staff learns, during the evaluation before admission, of previous precipitants to relapse. Learning the precipitants to relapse helps the patient avoid known noxious situations that are avoidable and helps the patient prepare carefully for situations that are unavoidable. This again is part of educating the patient in self-care—avoidance of that which can be avoided and preparation for that which cannot. Furthermore, it should be noted that in a community residence there is close staff contact with the patient, placing the staff in a position to observe signs of unexpected strengths in the patient. These signs then can be exploited in a positive way, bringing a new mastery of another sort to the patient.

The traditional community residence embodied in the long-term group residence has an ideology that differs from that of the hospital. In contrast to the hospital, the community residence is conceived of as being small, family modeled, integrated within the community, and an open society, whereas the hospital is seen as large, medically modeled, isolated from the community, and a closed society (Budson 1978). In particular, the "family-modeled social system" is the ideological basis for all phases of the community residence's life. This means, for example, that the community of patients is involved in decision making in the facility—from choosing wallpaper and fabrics in decorating the house, to selecting foods, to choosing weekend activities, to deciding details of house policies. Participation gives patients an opportunity to have the beneficial experience of decision making, which is a preparation for independent living. Allowing patients to make decisions about the community residence contrasts with hospital practices; hospitals usually keep patients very remote from decision making regarding the hospital ward, which is the patients' milieu. The staff of the community residence is small, stable, and committed to this patient-participation philosophy. In any community residence, staff act as role models because they tend to be more stable figures than are found on a hospital ward, and at the same time they are more open to, and seen as "real people" by, the residents of the facility.

Much of the therapeutic work done in the community residence helps the patient to come to terms with the devastating nature of the illness of schizophrenia and to make a positive adjustment to it. First, the patient must accept the illness and the usefulness of medication to help control its symptoms. Next, the patient must engage in mourning the lost ego-ideal. The patient often goes through a secondary depression at this point. Tricyclic antidepressants may be helpful adjunct therapy at this stage. Next, on resolution of the depression, Choras (personal communication, 1994) described a need for the development of ego compromises. Now the patient comes to terms with what he or she can realistically do. Vocational rehabilitation is an important component at this stage of treatment. Vocational evaluation and careful placement in a sheltered work setting can be crucial in helping to build new self-esteem. The final rehabilitative stage is described as the testing of the new ego-ideal. Here the patient adjusts to a newfound success. Often, such success frightens the patient, who feels it to be commensurate with abandonment. Reassurance from the milieu helps the working through at this stage.

Patients leave the residence after varying lengths of stay when they have acquired sufficient life skills within the program so that they are judged to be able to manage their lives in a more independent setting. More often than not, this means a move to a cooperative apartment program.

The high-expectation transitional halfway house is used to care for some of the healthiest patients, increasing their capacity to function in the community. However, more patients are going to these facilities after only 1 or 2 weeks of hospitalization, and their illnesses are, in fact, often quite acute. A significant difference from patients in the long-term group residence is that patients in the high-expectation halfway house usually have a mood disorder instead of psychosis, so there is an inherent higher level of functioning in patients. As a homelike residential bridge preparing a patient for independent living, this transitional facility offers life skills development through shared household responsibilities such as menu planning, cooking, and personal quarters upkeep. In addition, this facility provides a weekly program of large- and small-group meetings in the evening, individual case management, and assistance in implementing a meaningful 30-hour-per-week activity program outside of the house consisting of work, school, or a psychiatric day program. Unique in the staffing of the high-expectation halfway house is a live-in person who makes the facility his or her primary domicile; this permits him or her to become a true role-model figure. The live-in staff person is supplemented during the late afternoon by counselors and professional clinicians, depending on the size of the program. The halfway house is usually located off the hospital grounds and is best sited in an urban area close to public transportation and first-level job opportunities such as fast-food restaurants, shops, and stores.

Central to this milieu of patients, who are healthier than those of the two programs discussed previously, is the ideal of fostering continual self-discovery and mastery of self-care. This usually means learning about one's vulnerabilities and one's strengths, and learning how to minimize the former and enhance the latter to preserve health. The concept of altruism is stressed in the milieu, which in this context means caring about fellow house residents. Caring fosters true social relationships that in turn foster an extended psychosocial kinship system (Budson and Jolley 1978). This social network of patients can help foster mutual caring among friends, which can have a profound effect in helping patients to stay well. As a result of all this education in the milieu, patients are prepared to note adverse changes in their friends and are able to act on these observations either by intervening themselves or by calling for help.

A type of interpersonal dynamic characteristically seen in the halfway house can be put to good clinical use. Within the context of the social matrix of the program, a patient, often without being aware, repeats characteristic, stereotypical relationship patterns reflecting family patterns that have detrimentally distorted his or her life relationships. For example, staff of the community residence are often experienced as and reacted to as parental figures. Fellow residents are experienced as and reacted to as siblings. Sibling rivalries and jealousies; raging, distrustful, and paranoid attitudes toward parents; and playing off one parent against another, often in characteristic sexual patterns, with one idealized and one demeaned—all are played out with house staff and residents. In this situation, the staff has a golden opportunity to interpret these reactions and to elucidate the nature of the distortions. House meetings with fellow residents can be instrumental in clarifying the distorted views a frightened, distrustful, or angry resident may have adopted. In the community residence, the patient is given a real opportunity to find a new lifestyle liberated from old patterns.

The length of stay may vary depending on both the clinical task at hand and on the limitations enforced by managed care companies. For some patients who have significant characterological deficits, a 4-month stay enables significant rehabilitative gains. Time will then have been provided for working on the newly developed self, for working through new relationships with the family, and for developing new life and work skills.

For other patients, a shorter stay can at least provide initial stability to a stormy clinical situation, as well as a consultation to the referring care providers to help develop a new care plan that focuses on patients' continued clinical progress on discharge.

The cooperative apartment provides the most independent living situation of all community residences for mentally ill persons. The cooperative apartment aims to provide as much independent living as possible while providing support, supervision, and structure that can make all the difference between successful community tenure and relapse. In this program, residents must have the life skills to take responsibility for themselves in shopping, cooking, paying for utilities, and handling neighbor relations—all of the issues that independent living entails. The staffing is usually only one social worker or other clinician supervising each two-family unit, which houses eight residents. The program includes ongoing individual case management as required and several community/apartment meetings to assist residents in learning how to live together. The apartment program treats patients who have psychiatric illnesses at various severity levels. The critical issue is the capability of the patient to function appropriately in the community with only minimal staff supervision. Thus, there may be a delusional schizophrenic patient who, at the same time, has all of his or her life skills and the capacity to contain his or her actions so that they are appropriate. Staff are always available by electronic page.

Some Generic Clinical Features of Community Residential Care

In the previous section, some program-specific clinical considerations were described. The following discussion addresses additional clinical features that are generally applicable to patients in various programs, with the possible exception of the acute residence, in which there may not be sufficient time for all of the features to find full expression.

Evaluation at Admission

Significant members of the referring and receiving units should be present for the intake evaluation. Disagreements among the staff involved in evaluating and managing the patient should be aired at this time. Disagreements often are a sign of diagnostic ambiguity, and they can lead to further diagnostic clarification in the new setting. Critical issues to be discussed include psychiatric and medical history of the patient, current pharmacological regimen and rationale, dynamics of the current episode, family's relationship with the patient, planned milieu program for the patient, evaluation of the patient's strengths and life skills levels, anticipated length of stay and ultimate disposition, and planned inpatient backup if needed. Disqualifying conditions include lack of control of destructive impulses to the self,

others, or property; ongoing substance abuse; sexual promiscu-
ity that is out of control; and habitual lying.

Elements of the Clinical Program

Experience with patients in the community residential setting
has shown that double bedrooms are preferred rather than sin-
gles. Living with roommates facilitates socialization and creates
a "buddy" system, making the residence a safer place. Furthermore, roommates, over time, increasingly tend to look after each
other's well-being. For example, a resident will come to the staff
if it is felt that the roommate is in some secret difficulty. The
problems can range from suicidal feelings, to drug problems, to
avoiding the daily program, to some significant personal loss.
Double occupancy, then, provides checks and balances with regard to the clinical program and its behavioral codes, helping
prevent illicit drinking, sex, drugs, or antisocial behavior.

When the resident first moves in, the responsible clinician
makes a serious effort to form a strong therapeutic alliance by
getting to know the resident well. The likelihood of a good outcome is enhanced by the quality of this alliance. In collaboration
with the patient, a problem list is developed that identifies all of
the resident's deficiencies, followed by specific therapeutic measures designed to correct them. As appropriate, schedules for
life skills development are drawn up, or outside activity schedules are identified. The resident's share in domestic chores is
identified and described. A schedule of weekly individual sessions with clinicians is identified also.

The house meeting can be viewed as a paradigm of the clinical program and is included in the routine of all facilities. These
meetings can be important therapeutic events in several ways.
First, each patient, despite his or her shyness or isolation, is
afforded an opportunity to speak about meaningful issues with
the entire group. Second, through the feedback the patient receives from fellow residents, it is discovered that he or she is not
so strange, nor is his or her problem so unique: the patient is
not alone. Third, through the help of housemates, the resident

over time learns how to talk about his or her problems, and eventually the discussions help him or her effectively master the problems. Each person's sharing diminishes isolation, enhances self-understanding, promotes accessibility, and undermines paranoia. Each gain for the individual carries a reciprocal gain for the entire group. Openness on the part of both the individual and group facilitates a mutuality, a closeness, and a common helping and support that carry into the milieu, beyond the limits of the house meeting. This effect, too, is reciprocal: group solidarity and increasing pride in the milieu foster a feeling of strength and capacity in the group to do further meaningful work.

Leaving the Community Residence

The resident should depart, if at all possible, to a living situation within the context of an existing social network. Ex-residents should move into a living arrangement with known others, such as former housemates, and should not live alone. A daily program of familiar activities should be in place. A therapeutic relationship with a significant trusted other, often a clinician, to whom the patient can turn in time of trouble is the sine qua non of requirements for departure. The medication regimen should be stabilized and provisions made for medical monitoring where appropriate. Ideally, the ex-resident's relationship with his or her family is also under control so that pathological family patterns will not reemerge without some provision for checking them and preventing relapse. Finally, it has been found that a continuing relationship with the community residence, through an ex-resident program and personal ties to the facility, is desirable. It is apparent that the resident moving out benefits from the greatest amount of stability and resources as possible.

Conclusion

Community residential care is a significant component of the continuum of mental health services because it fosters a more complete rehabilitative result than is possible in the inpatient hospital alone. It permits more time for stabilization of the patient biologically, psychosocially, and psychologically and often lends opportunity for genuine human growth before the patient reenters independent living in the community. It is both humane and cost-effective. Ideally, community residential care is a critical service keeping the hope alive that mental health services in the future can still meet the traditional ancient altruistic goals of health care.

References

Budson RD: The psychiatric halfway house. Psychiatric Annals 6:64–83, 1973

Budson RD: The Psychiatric Halfway House: A Handbook of Theory and Practice. Pittsburgh, PA, University of Pittsburgh Press, 1978

Budson RD: Sheltered housing for the mentally ill: an overview. McLean Hospital Journal 4:140–157, 1979

Budson RD: Models of supportive living: community residential care, in Handbook of Schizophrenia, Vol 4: Psychosocial Treatment of Schizophrenia. Edited by Herz MI, Keith SJ, Docherty JP. Amsterdam, The Netherlands, Elsevier Science, 1990, pp 317–338

Budson RD: Community residential and partial hospital care: low-cost alternative systems in the spectrum of care. Psychiatr Q 65:209–220, 1994

Budson RD, Jolley RE: A crucial factor in community program success: the extended psychosocial kinship system. Schizophr Bull 4:609–621, 1978

Glasscote RM, Gudeman JE, Elpers R: Halfway Houses for the Mentally Ill. Washington, DC, Joint Information Service of the American Psychiatric Association and the National Association for Mental Health, 1971

Landy D, Greenblatt M: Halfway House. Washington, DC, U.S. Department of Health, Education, and Welfare, Vocational Rehabilitation Administration, 1965

Raush HL, Raush CL: The Halfway House Movement: A Search for Sanity. New York, Appleton-Century-Crofts, 1968

6 Partial Hospital Care

Laurel J. Kiser, Ph.D., M.B.A.
David B. Pruitt, M.D.

Along the continuum of ambulatory behavioral health care, partial hospital services represent the most intensive level of care providing crisis stabilization and acute symptom reduction (Kiser et al. 1993). Partial hospital care is often used as an alternative to inpatient care, as a prevention for hospital care, and as a transitional setting to shorten a hospital stay. Partial hospitalization means "a time-limited, ambulatory, active treatment program that offers therapeutically intensive, coordinated, structured clinical services within a stable therapeutic milieu to persons with severe psychiatric disorders" (Block and Lefkovitz 1991, p. 2).

It is 1:00 P.M. Friday. The telephone rings. The behavioral health care system intake coordinator answers and takes information about an emergency admission. The intake coordinator schedules an interview for 3:00 P.M.

At approximately 3:05 P.M., Ms. J arrives for her appointment accompanied by her mother. Ms. J is a 23-year-old white female. She is well groomed, although pale and tense looking. She sits quietly without making eye contact. Her mother does most of the talking.

She presents her daughter's story: Ms. J attended high school and 2 years of college. Life seemed to be going well until her junior year when she began to have trouble concentrating, difficulty sleeping, frequent crying spells, and angry outbursts. Although she sought outpatient treatment, she failed to complete the school year and moved back home. Over the past 2 years, she has had difficulty holding jobs due to recurring problems with depression. Continued therapy and several medication trials did little to stabilize her mood. Her mother reports that both her paternal grandfather and maternal uncle suffered from depression.

Over the last few weeks, her symptoms have escalated to the point where she is verbally threatening her younger sister and also is talking about suicide. When she talks about suicide, she contemplates taking pills or drowning herself. She is not eating regularly and has lost 7 pounds in the past month.

After assessing for suicidal risk and availability of family supports, the decision is made to admit Ms. J to partial hospital services. The intake clinician, Ms. J, and her mother, in collaboration with the attending psychiatrist, develop the initial treatment plan detailing coverage for the weekend. This plan includes Ms. J's signing a no-harm contract, arrangements for family support and supervision, and periodic check-ins by the on-call crisis team.

A 3-week stay in the partial hospital service included twice-weekly individual therapy, daily group therapies, specialty groups, and structured peer activities. Family therapy sessions occurred weekly. Therapeutic assignments involved initiating weekend plans with friends, visiting a college counselor to investigate returning to school, and keeping a mood journal. Ms. J started on fluoxetine hydrochloride 20 mg every morning, beginning on the second day of treatment in the program.

Ms. J experienced several difficult days during her first week in treatment. Before leaving the program on those days, she was evaluated by the medical director to determine suicidal intent. The program staff notified her parents of her increased risk and made plans for monitoring her condition during the evening. Telemonitoring was used to assess her condition hourly, with the on-call staff monitoring her responses and ready to assist her if necessary.

At discharge, Ms. J had gone without suicidal thoughts for 5 days. Although still expressing some problems sleeping and doubts about peer relations, she reported improved mood, concentration, and appetite. Aftercare plans involved continuation in individual and group therapy, part-time attendance at the community college, and continuation on her antidepressant medication.

Staff Composition

Staffing Patterns and Ratios

A multidisciplinary staff composes the treatment team for most partial hospital programs. The disciplines represented are psychiatry, psychology, social work, counseling, nursing, occupational therapy, recreational therapy, education, and other physical health disciplines. Most programs use master's-level counselors, social workers, and bachelor's-level mental health workers as core full-time staff.

Several staffing patterns are common to partial hospital programs. Some programs are staffed based on traditional hospital models where nursing plays a pivotal role in managing the milieu. Other programs rely more heavily on occupational, educational or vocational, recreational, and activity therapists to direct day-to-day programming.

Partial hospital staffing can be accomplished using either an open or closed staff model. In open staff models, it is important that a core treatment staff is identified that includes professionals who are consistently available to patients. Closed staff models with salaried professionals offer some advantages, especially the ability to develop an integrated clinical team. This closed staffing model also may be particularly advantageous for systems interested in going at risk financially.

Partial hospital care provides intensive therapeutic services for patients with acute, unstable conditions and must be staffed accordingly. Experienced clinical staff and low staff-to-patient ratios are necessary. Staff-to-patient ratios recommended in the standards and guidelines for partial hospitalization suggest that staff numbers be based on the needs of the patient group treated in terms of age, level of functioning, and severity of psychiatric symptoms (Block and Lefkovitz 1991).

Staff Roles

Leadership roles in partial hospital services are critical to the success of the milieu. Programs need to have a program director who is on site daily and in charge of day-to-day operations. This individual needs to have the appropriate education and clinical experience to deal with the specific needs of the target patient population.

The role of the medical personnel in terms of leadership is also important. Partial hospital services, offering intense treatment in lieu of inpatient care, require consistent medical leadership. Staffing at this level of care incorporates a medical director who supervises patient care and is ultimately responsible for all clinical services provided (Kiser et al. 1993).

Staff Satisfaction

Working within a partial hospital setting can be tremendously rewarding and tremendously stressful. Thus, monitoring staff satisfaction is a critical administrative responsibility. Both individual job functioning and satisfaction and team functioning and satisfaction deserve attention. Combating staff burnout is an ongoing challenge. Building a culture with a shared, qualitative value system that supports the philosophy of ambulatory care, communication among disciplines, and commitment to patient wellness and empowerment is essential.

Target Population

Admission and Discharge Criteria

Admission criteria for partial hospital services (Table 6–1) mark the boundaries between patients that can be safely treated in an ambulatory setting and those who require 24-hour care. To address this issue adequately, admission criteria focus on level of previous intervention, level of functioning, severity of psychiatric symptoms, behavior control, suicidal or homicidal potential, alcohol and drug involvement, and physical health. As patients in ambulatory settings often need to rely on family and community supports to augment treatment, admission criteria for partial hospital care include an assessment of these resources. Overlapping the support system criteria with the patient criteria determines a patient's ability to use and benefit from treatment within an ambulatory treatment setting. Finally, the patient's ability to pay must be considered.

Patient Access to Services

To respond effectively to patients in crisis, partial hospital services must have intake and admission processes that respond immediately to patients' needs. A patient requiring the level of intensity offered by partial hospital care should have access to services within 24 hours of initial contact (Kiser et al. 1993). Partial hospital services that do not operate 7 days a week need a system for providing clinical coverage to patients who are admitted to the service late in the day or on the weekend.

Discharge Planning

Discharge planning is an integral part of all treatment planning within partial hospital services. Discharge planning begins during the initial intake and continues throughout the treatment process as discharge goals are formulated and clarified. During treatment, the treatment team continually monitors progress toward discharge goals with participation from the patient and family and, ever increasingly, from the managed care intermediary.

Discharge planning within partial hospital services is dictated by the following principle: patients receive treatment in the least restrictive environment that provides the structure and intensity necessary for the shortest time possible to reach maximum treatment benefit. To accomplish this, discharge planning is done in a manner that maximizes a successful transition to the patient's new treatment setting (either more or less structured). Thus discharge planning involves attention to issues of termination, liaison with community resources (e.g., residential set-

Table 6–1.   Admission criteria for partial hospital care

Criteria	Descriptions
Previous treatment	Sufficient trial of outpatient/intensive outpatient care without response; severity of symptoms and level of functioning require intensive intervention despite previous treatment
Level of functioning	Marked impairment in multiple areas of daily functioning, especially in work or school
Severity of symptoms	Acute disabling symptoms related to an emerging condition or exacerbation of a severe/persistent disorder
Behavior control	Ability to control, on a limited basis, impulses and behavior
Suicidal/homicidal intent	Risk factors and protective factors are balanced so as not to require 24-hour confinement
Alcohol and drug involvement	Does not require 24-hour/day medical care for detoxification
Physical health	Does not require 24-hour/day medical care
Ability to pay	Patient or family has the resources to support treatment

tings, work or school settings), development of aftercare treatment plans, and follow-up strategies that encourage compliance with aftercare recommendations.

Census Issues

Referrals

Traditionally, partial hospital patients have come in equal numbers from inpatient and outpatient providers. This is probably still the referral base for partial hospital services within hospital systems. For freestanding programs, this is no longer necessarily true. As many hospital-based systems develop aftercare programs that include a day component, referrals to freestanding programs have decreased. To maintain an inpatient referral base, freestanding partial hospital services need actively to pursue networking opportunities and cooperative relationships with inpatient services.

Fluctuations

Census fluctuations are a natural part of operating a partial hospital service, especially for child and adolescent providers. Drops in patient numbers occur regularly during the early summer, early fall, and surrounding the holidays. Management of staffing patterns and operational budgets during low-census times is a challenge for partial hospital providers.

Diagnosis and Treatment

Assessment and Diagnosis

The assessment process begins with an evaluation of need for treatment and determination of the appropriate level of care.

For partial hospital care, this initial assessment must focus on evaluating the individual patient's personality dynamics, target symptoms, level of impulse control, and the availability and reliability of family and community support systems.

After determining the patient's appropriateness for partial hospital care and admission to the program, a comprehensive biopsychosocial assessment is necessary. This assessment needs to be coordinated with previous evaluations, if available, from other services or episodes of care.

An assessment in a partial hospital program is multidisciplinary and needs to include an evaluation of functioning in the following areas: emotional, cognitive, behavioral, social, recreational, daily living, educational/vocational, legal, medical/physical, and familial. A thorough patient and family history of previous mental illness and substance use/abuse is important, as is an inventory of previous treatments. Documentation of the need for a history and physical examination is necessary. If a history and physical are needed, these procedures can be performed within the service or a referral can be made to a community physician.

To provide the most effective treatment planning, assessment within community-based, ambulatory mental health programs, such as partial hospitalization, incorporates an evaluation of patient and family strengths, limitations, and resources. Use of multiple sources of information and observations improves the validity of assessment within a partial hospital program. Gathering pertinent information from community sources, such as employers or teachers, is necessary for planning effective interventions within the multimodal structure of partial hospital care.

Assessment findings are integrated into a summary that describes the patient, the illness, and the objectives for treatment. A comprehensive biopsychosocial formulation of the patient and the current illness leads to a diagnosis based on DSM-IV (American Psychiatric Association 1994). An initial assessment of aftercare needs is also formulated. This comprehensive assessment does not end the evaluation phase of treatment. Assessment, to be most effective, is an ongoing process, with observations of the patient within the milieu and structured treatment settings used continually as input in treatment planning.

Program of Therapeutic Activities

Partial hospital services offer a multimodal approach to treatment. The program of therapeutic activities offered is based on an individual treatment plan that outlines specific problems, objectives, and treatment modalities prescribed. A patient's treatment plan directs the patient's movement through the daily schedule of therapeutic activities and also addresses the need for community involvement and liaison with other necessary support systems.

Active therapies.   Active treatment constitutes the majority of program hours and includes group psychotherapy, psychoeducational activities, adjunctive and life skills groups, individual therapy, and medication evaluation and management. Observation of the patient in every aspect of the program and reports obtained regarding participation within the home and community provide a wealth of information that can be used in therapy. This comprehensive information base allows the therapeutic experiences in partial hospital care to be different from outpatient or inpatient psychotherapies. Active therapies in partial hospital services use material from daily encounters with families, parents, children or siblings, peers and relatives, staff, and other patients to address dysfunction in these systemic areas.

Therapeutic milieu.   An active, highly structured therapeutic milieu is the backbone of most partial hospital care. What makes up a therapeutic milieu? In a partial hospital service, look for coordinated, connected therapeutic activities; dedicated, adequate space and furnishings; continuity of staffing patterns; and active involvement of patients in the therapeutic community.

Beyond designing a therapeutic milieu within the program, partial hospital care also focuses on restructuring patients' milieu within the family, work, school, and community. This is a necessary requirement and therapeutic advantage for modalities that offer intense treatment without 24-hour-a-day confinement.

Occupational training/schooling.   Patients in partial hospital care often have regressed functioning in work or school. To develop strategies to reestablish and improve skills in these areas, partial hospital services offer therapeutic experiences that stress occupational or educational skills. This preparation for return to work or school is an important treatment objective. To facilitate return to work or school, schedules of attendance in partial hospital services may be adjusted to allow gradual return to these activities, such as attendance for half days or 2–3 days a week. Afternoon and evening programming may allow a patient to resume normal educational/vocational activity while continuing to receive intensive treatment.

Family involvement.   The standards and guidelines for partial hospitalization recommend that families are actively involved in the treatment process (Block and Lefkovitz 1991; Block et al. 1991). This involvement, when possible, extends from initial evaluation of family functioning and resources to measurement of family satisfaction with treatment following discharge. Using a broad-based definition of family to include the patient's biological family, custodian, and significant others, partial hospital services structure opportunities for active treatment experiences that include relevant family members whenever clinically indicated.

Program extenders.   An important feature of partial hospital services is integration of available community services and supports into the treatment plan and process. Early in the treatment process, therapists begin encouraging patients and their families to become actively involved in community activities and groups as a part of their treatment so that participation with these community supports is firmly established at the time of discharge. Active community liaison with these other providers, agencies, and self-help groups by partial hospital staff increases the effectiveness of these interventions and the generalization of treatment gains following discharge.

Special treatment procedures and emergency coverage. Treatment of patients with suicidal/homicidal ideation and behavior, aggressivity, and so on challenges partial hospital care as an alternative to inpatient care. To treat severely disturbed, and sometimes dangerous, patients without the locked doors and other safeguards of inpatient care, partial hospital services establish highly structured routines and special treatment policies. Procedures designed to manage crises and ensure patient safety within partial hospital services must address the same set of behaviors as those encountered by inpatient services yet must offer different therapeutic responses.

Special treatment procedures designed for use in partial hospital settings rely on firm expectations for patient compliance with programmatic rules, augmentation of the structure of normal living arrangements by providing supervision and additional support, and increased therapeutic vigilance by clinical staff both during and after program hours. Telemonitoring technologies are valuable resources for extending the ability of partial care providers to maintain patients within the home/community environment.

Partial hospital services treat patients with unstable and severe psychiatric disorders; some will not be able to function adequately within an ambulatory structure. Therefore, all programs need crisis management services that meet the requirements described. Partial hospital services incorporate an on-call system staffed by clinicians who have immediate access to information regarding current clinical and treatment status. This service provides support and guidance during crises, encourages use of problem-solving skills, and attempts to enhance patients' and families' competence in crisis resolution. When appropriate, the on-call service also facilitates admission to 23-hour observation beds, crisis stabilization beds, or an inpatient unit. This on-call system includes backup by a psychiatrist. Finally, to facilitate emergency inpatient admissions, partial hospital services maintain an established affiliation with both a general and psychiatric hospital.

Space and Props

Sites

Partial hospital services take place in a variety of organizational settings, with 40% of programs operating as part of multiservice mental health organizations, another 40% operating as part of general or psychiatric hospitals, about 8% freestanding (Culhane et al. 1994), and the remainder operating in other sites. The sites for partial hospital services can be multiple locations, and, although the name implies hospital-based programming, the site for care is often a freestanding building away from hospital grounds. Placement of partial hospital services away from hospital grounds has the advantage of diluting the possible stigma associated with psychiatric hospital care. It may have the disadvantage of inefficient use of space. Some regulatory agencies and payers, such as Civilian Health and Medical Programs for the Uniformed Services (CHAMPUS), require partial hospital services to occupy separate and dedicated space.

Geographic distance between the program site and the target patient population base is a major issue, as is easy access to the available space. Because patients must come and go every day, facilitating this access is essential, such as providing adequate parking and transportation to and from the program. Multisite services are also increasing in popularity to help ease access.

Physical Plant Requirements

State, local, and national regulatory agencies provide some guidelines regarding physical plant requirements that must be met before licensing the facility. On a practical level, designing space for partial hospital services involves providing sufficient space for the target census numbers and for the daily programming plans. Besides the space required for active therapies, space for practice of daily living skills, including a kitchen, a room for recreational activities, a classroom, and a vocational workshop, needs to be accessible. Estimates of minimum space requirements range from 150 square feet per patient for adult services to 200 square feet per patient for child and adolescent providers. All space, design, and furnishings should address the needs of target patient groups, especially their developmental factors. For instance, services designed for young children need to be located on the ground floor, need bathroom facilities scaled appropriately, and need small-sized, highly durable furnishings and play equipment. Facilities for geriatric patients may require proximity to medical services and should be designed for the physical, behavioral, and cognitive needs of this special population.

There are other practical considerations for space design within partial hospital services. In planning space for partial hospital care, ensuring visual access between open areas and activity areas can be helpful in allowing staff to monitor patient activity in several locations simultaneously. An additional space consideration for managing patient behavior is seclusion rooms. For the most part, partial hospital facilities do not include seclusion rooms with restraint equipment; however, quiet spaces where a distraught, disruptive patient can be removed from the milieu are crucial.

Unique Aspects of Partial Hospital Services

Partial hospital services represent a specific modality of care along the behavioral health care continuum. As such, there are both unique benefits and special challenges that affect this modality. Table 6–2 lists the unique benefits of partial hospitalization, and Table 6–3 presents the special challenges and problems.

Table 6–2.   Unique benefits of partial hospital services

Allows the patient with an acute psychiatric disorder to remain with his or her family and in the community while receiving intensive treatment.

Encourages the patient and family or support system to maintain responsibility while stabilizing the patient's condition and beginning the treatment process.

Provides at least 4 hours of daily service for the patient, thus lessening the burden for the family or support system for part of each day.

Can give the patient a break for part of each day from a dysfunctional family or support system and a chaotic, perhaps dangerous, environment.

Avoids/minimizes the potential iatrogenic effects that accompany institutional care, such as stigma, dependency, and loss of autonomy and independence.

Provides the freedom for patients to continue involvement in extracurricular activities, such as part-time work and social affairs.

Eases transitions from either less intensive or more intensive treatment.

Table 6–3.   Special challenges and problems of partial hospital providers

Manage severely disturbed patients in an ambulatory setting. Maintaining a balance between treatment in the least restrictive environment and safety is a primary consideration.

Manage census issues effectively, such as underutilization and daily attendance. The partial hospital modality has a history of underutilization, a problem that has resulted in the failure of many programs. In addition, helping patients with severe pathology attend treatment according to a prescribed schedule is also a challenge.

Manage the fiscal viability of an ambulatory behavioral health program. Reimbursement for partial hospitalization is only gradually increasing as payers move away from traditional indemnity plans that paid for either inpatient or outpatient care. However, profit margins for partial hospital services are *not* comparable to inpatient care, and organizations must adjust financial goals accordingly. Cost creep (gradual increases in the charges for partial hospital care), in an era of cost containment, is perhaps the most serious fiscal threat to a modality gaining in popularity.

Manage staff stress and burnout.

Facilitate patient access. As an ambulatory modality, the issue of geographical distance between the patient and the site of care needs to be considered. This is especially challenging in rural areas.

References

American Psychiatric Association: Diagnostic and Statistical Manual of Mental Disorders, 4th Edition. Washington, DC, American Psychiatric Association, 1994

Block B, Lefkovitz PM: Standards and Guidelines for Partial Hospitalization. Washington, DC, American Association for Partial Hospitalization, 1991

Block B, Arney K, Campbell D, et al: Standards and Guidelines for Child and Adolescent Partial Hospitalization. Washington, DC, American Association for Partial Hospitalization, 1991

Culhane DP, Hadley TR, Kiser LJ: A national profile of partial hospital programs. Continuum 1:81–94, 1994

Kiser LJ, Lefkovitz PM, Kennedy LL, et al: The continuum of ambulatory mental health services. Behavioral Healthcare Tomorrow 2:14–16, 1993

Additional Readings

Herz MI: Research overview in day treatment. International Journal of Partial Hospitalization 1:33–34, 1982

Hoge MA, Farrell SP, Munchel ME, et al: Therapeutic factors in partial hospitalization. Psychiatry 51:199–210, 1988

Lefkovitz PM: The short-term program, in Differing Approaches to Partial Hospitalization, Vol 38. Edited by Goldberg K. San Francisco, CA, Jossey-Bass, 1988, pp 31–49

Leibenluft E, Leibenluft RF: Reimbursement for partial hospitalization: a survey and policy implications. Am J Psychiatry 145:1514–1520, 1988

Rosie JS: Partial hospitalization: a review of recent literature. Hospital and Community Psychiatry 38:1291–1299, 1987

Wagner BD, Plotkin DA, Lefkovitz PM, et al: Standards and Guidelines for Geriatric Partial Hospitalization. Washington, DC, American Association for Partial Hospitalization, 1994

Zimet SG, Farley GK: Day treatment for children in the United States. Journal of American Academy of Child Psychiatry 24:732–738, 1985

7 Hospital-Based Alcohol and Drug Treatment

Richard J. Frances, M.D.
Evelyn Wilson, M.S.W.
Judith H. Wiegand, M.A.

Mr. M, a 42-year-old divorced former policeman and father of a 12-year-old girl, called the Hackensack University Medical Center's Addiction Treatment Center (New Jersey) for an appointment. He had lost his wife and job, could not stop drinking, and wanted to die. He has had an extensive history of heavy drinking that has led to unemployment and frequent feelings of depression with some suicidal ideation. Mr. M, who has consumed a quart of vodka a day since age 25, has had multiple failed attempts at treatment, including inpatient detoxification and rehabilitation due to years of denial and treatment resistance. His longest period of sobriety has been 9 months.

Only in the last year has he accepted his need to stop drinking and agreed to accept help. This came about after his divorce, which occurred 1 year after termination from the police force for drinking on the job, verbal abusiveness, and, on one occasion, participation in a brawl with a fellow

91

officer. Mr. M has been depressed, has felt hopeless about finding another job, has been unable to stop drinking, and has felt inadequate as a father. He has problems falling asleep at night without drinking, has early morning awakenings, and has a poor appetite. He has lost 10 pounds and has had episodes of severe alcohol withdrawal, including hearing voices, seeing things, and tremulousness, which at times have required benzodiazepines and hospitalization.

Mr. M is typical of patients with a dual psychiatric diagnosis (alcoholism and depression) who come to the Addiction Treatment Center. They are likely to require initial medically managed detoxification and careful psychiatric evaluation for 5–10 days on our inpatient general hospital psychiatric unit with an addiction service line. This should be followed by partial hospitalization for approximately 1 month, intensive outpatient treatment in the Addiction Treatment Center for another 12–16 weeks, then follow-up treatment. The specific length of stay is tailored to the individual case and is based on team decision and the biopsychosocial assessment of the patient. We follow Mr. M through the system as an example of how this is done.

In this chapter, we describe the design of the Addiction Treatment Center and the efforts to deliver excellent cost-effective psychiatric and chemical dependency care that maximizes each patient's and family's potential for self-esteem, self-care, and a healthy lifestyle. A comprehensive range of therapeutic services is offered at Hackensack University Medical Center as part of its general hospital service line in addiction psychiatry. The full spectrum of professionals, including psychiatrists, nurses, social workers, and alcoholism counselors, provides care in a variety of settings: a brief-stay inpatient general psychiatry unit, a partial hospitalization program that focuses on dual-diagnosis patients, an adolescent program, and an organized outpatient addiction psychiatry program that has the capacity to perform outpatient detoxification whenever indicated. The full range of the American Society of Addiction Medicine (ASAM) level 1–4 placement criteria is available. In this chapter, we do not provide a guideline but a model of biopsychosocial treatment for addicted patients.

In the managed care environment, there has been a trend toward shorter lengths of stay and a movement from models of long-term inpatient rehabilitation toward short, intermediate, and long-term measurable outpatient rehabilitation with decreased intensity. Programs are designed to serve managed care and capitated groups of patients and provide rapid intervention, availability of emergency care, comprehensive evaluation and diagnosis, early crisis intervention, individualized treatment protocols, clinical targeted outcomes, and follow-up care.

The foundations of treatment modalities are built on a biopsychosocial paradigm with an understanding of a strong hereditary component that can be affected by developmental, environmental, and cultural stressors. The treatment approach is tailored to each patient's disorder, level of function and disability, and specific psychosocial needs. The biopsychosocial model promotes continuity of care that emphasizes the least restrictive alternative and the most cost-effective service to the individual and the individual's family. Families are heavily involved in the treatment program. A general hospital with strong outpatient programs can provide medical and inpatient backup support while keeping the patient functioning and receiving treatment out of the hospital and in the community. This is the model also used to instruct rotations of residents from our affiliate, the Department of Psychiatry, University of Medicine and Dentistry of New Jersey—New Jersey Medical School.

Because Mr. M requires inpatient treatment with medically administered detoxification and psychiatric evaluation on the basis of suicidal ideation, severe alcohol withdrawal marked by hallucinations, elevated temperature and pulse, and tremulousness, he is admitted to a 24-bed inpatient unit. He meets the ASAM placement criteria for level 1, or medically supervised detoxification in a hospital. Both voluntary and involuntary patients are admitted to the inpatient unit. Our hospital unit provides a full range of acute treatment services, with a service line that focuses on dual-diagnosis patients. A full range of group and therapeutic modalities is available to structure a specific program for Mr. M, detoxify him, help him clearly see his diagnosis, help confront his denial, and prepare him to continue his recovery plan. In Mr. M's case, his severe withdrawal symptoms took 5 days to abate. At first thought to be substance induced, his major depression, including suicidal ideation, decreased somewhat by day 10. At that point, he began to feel hopeful about starting the partial hospital program and met with staff from there and was transferred. He continued in the partial hospital program for 5 hours per day, but his depression persisted. He was started on 20 mg of fluoxetine hydrochloride by day 14 because he stopped showing improvement, had persistent sleep problems, had poor self-esteem, and had difficulty getting himself into the program. The issue of when to start medication depends on making a diagnosis of an independent depression.

He did not drink in the partial hospital program and stayed for 25 days. His sleep had improved, his motivation for staying sober was taking hold, and he was ready for the intensive outpatient program. There he explored the triggers to relapse and ways to widen his social support system. He became engaged in nightly Alcoholics Anonymous (AA) attendance, had his medication monitored, and developed a solid therapeutic relationship with his certified addiction counselor. He dealt with important issues, including the need to find a new career as a security guard and how to improve his relationship with his daughter and former wife. He stayed in this program for 15 weeks. By week 15, his AA participation and work with a sponsor solidified, he began a new job, and he was ready for aftercare.

The Addiction Treatment Center is a comprehensive outpatient substance abuse program serving adults within the tristate area. This 3-hour-a-day structured program consists of group therapy, focus groups, daily or weekly individual or family therapy, and therapeutic education. The programs dispense a range of services, including ambulatory detoxification, intensive treatment, and partial hospitalization. By the time Mr. M left the partial hospital program, he had medical detoxification, had started taking antidepressant medication, and had psychiatric treatment for his additional diagnosis of major affective disorder. Once he arrived in the Addiction Treatment Center, he was not placed on the general track, but on the track for dual-diagnosis patients, which furnished greater attention from a psychiatrist than ordinarily is provided for garden-variety addictions. Treating depression and addiction increased the probability for favorable results and restored him to a better level of functioning than past treatment protocols. For adults, there is medical backup from the medical clinic; in the adolescent substance abuse program, a pediatrician is available on site. A crucial part of the program is involvement in the 12-Step program, and its philosophy is integrated into all treatment modalities. Mr. M was required to attend at least five 12-Step meetings each week.

Magnitude of the Problem

Alcoholism and drug abuse constitute the nation's number one public health problem and present a major challenge in designing and providing cost-effective services to a general hospital population. Studies have found that anywhere between 25% and 50% of patients who come to a general hospital have an additional alcohol and drug problem. In 1990, the economic costs of substance abuse to the country were estimated at $98.6 billion for alcohol abuse and $66.9 billion for drug abuse. Smoking costs were estimated at $72 billion. Males are three times more likely to be heavy drinkers and twice as likely to use marijuana frequently. Substance abuse patients are likely to have a number of relapses and may require repeated treatment geared toward relapse prevention. Compared with treatment for other chronic illnesses, treatment for alcoholism and drug abuse is more cost-effective; however, there is considerable denial among those with alcohol and drug problems. Many young people do not believe that heavy use is terribly dangerous and feel hopeless about treatment outcomes. There tends to be a progressive development of substance abuse problems, and by eighth grade, 70% of adolescents have consumed alcohol, 44% have smoked cigarettes, 10% have used marijuana, and 2% have tried cocaine. More than 500,000 or one-fourth of all deaths can be linked to nicotine, alcohol, and drug problems, with the lion's share related to nicotine addiction.

Alcoholism and drug abuse tend to be hereditary and familial illnesses, with approximately 40% of the population exposed to an alcoholic family member or a problem drinker in the family. Problems with alcohol and drug abuse are enormously costly to families, not only in terms of money spent on alcohol, cigarettes, and drugs, but also because of increased health-related costs, lost time from work, and legal consequences of addiction. People are often coerced into treatment by the workplace, families, and physicians; however, treatment outcome does not appear to be related to whether patients come in willingly or are coerced. Rather, risk factors such as having a positive family history of alcoholism, not holding a stable job, not having a family or support system, having more severe psychiatric illness, having an antisocial personality, and having a history of lack of success in periods of sobriety are negative prognostic factors. The reverse generally predicts a favorable outcome.

Addiction Treatment Service Line at Hackensack University Medical Center

A description of the addiction treatment services is provided in the remainder of this chapter, including the addiction treatment component of the general hospital inpatient unit, the Addiction Treatment Center, and the Adolescent Drug and Alcohol Prevention and Treatment program. The goals of the inpatient addiction treatment program are complete medical detoxification and evaluation, stabilization, and early treatment of additional psychiatric and medical problems.

The objectives of the inpatient program are to stabilize the presenting problems medically, educate the patient, medicate dual-diagnosis patients, increase compliance, reduce side effects, and provide the patient with a treatment plan that the patient can realistically utilize to continue the recovery process.

Criteria for inpatient admission to our psychiatric unit are based on ASAM and Coalition Universal Placement criteria and promote treatment matching. Patients must meet two or more of the following criteria:

- Patient meets DSM-IV (American Psychiatric Association 1994) criteria for substance-related disorders with intoxication or withdrawal.
- Patient may have a concurrent DSM-IV psychiatric disorder or medical condition with severity requiring admission.
- Patient is a relapsing patient with a history of delirium tremens, morning shakes, or convulsions.
- Patient has an addiction history indicating multiple drug abuse, including alcohol, requiring medical treatment in an acute-care setting.
- Patient's presenting symptoms and behavior indicate a complex mixture of psychiatric and addiction disorders requiring treatment in an acute-care setting.
- Patient has not accepted or has failed at less restrictive options, lacks social support, and requires a recovery environment.

The method of treatment to ease patients through the detoxification process is 24-hour clinical management with a team approach. After 24 hours, or when the patient becomes mentally clear, the patient receives a biopsychosocial and family evaluation and begins to participate in therapeutic activities. The patient learns about AA, Cocaine Anonymous, Narcotics Anonymous (NA), and other 12-Step programs with psychoeducation and therapy and participates in group therapy. A treatment plan is fully developed within 24 hours of the psychosocial evaluation. The structure of daily therapeutic activities includes medication evaluation as required; lectures; occupational, individual, and group therapy; and evaluation of medical complications. Currently, the average length of stay for substance abuse patients is 3–5 days, with a trend toward fewer days and continuing detoxification in the partial hospitalization program; however, patients with a dual diagnosis remain on the unit an average of 8.5 days. The therapeutic focus is aimed at developing skills for maintaining sobriety and preventing relapse. Treatment plans are designed to promote self-esteem, self-worth, and self-care, and patients are motivated to continue the recovery process.

Discharge criteria for the inpatient unit include completion of the objectives of the treatment plan: patients are no longer in danger of withdrawal, are no longer suicidal or homicidal, and are ready for outpatient treatment. Completion of medical detoxification is evidenced by improved physical health. At any given time, 4–10 patients on the 24-bed general psychiatric inpatient unit are part of this service line. Several nurses take responsibility for staff in-service training and for the structured program of addiction lectures and study groups for patients.

Addiction Treatment Center at Hackensack University Medical Center

The outpatient Addiction Treatment Center has approximately 30,000 visits per year and is the largest of the outpatient programs in the Department of Psychiatry. The program principally serves a middle- and lower-class population in the Bergen County, New Jersey, area, which includes a wide range of occupations, ethnic groups, ages, and referral sources. The center offers a variety of services, including biopsychosocial assessment and evaluation, individual counseling and therapy, group therapy, family and couples therapy, crisis and family intervention, ambulatory medical detoxification (alcohol and most drugs), partial hospitalization, adolescent intensive outpatient treatment, a dual-diagnosis program, women's and men's programs, an aftercare program, an adult children of alcoholics program, and an intoxicated drivers' resource center educational group.

Ambulatory Detoxification Program in a Partial Hospital

The goal of the ambulatory detoxification program is for the patient to complete an initial phase of detoxification as an outpatient in approximately 2–8 days (average 5) and participate in a plan for continued treatment to alter the course of the disease. The program's objectives are to stabilize the patient medically, begin to educate the patient about the disease of alcoholism and drug abuse, motivate the patient to maintain sobriety and continue recovery treatment, and provide a treatment plan that the patient can realistically use to continue recovery and prevent relapse. The admission criteria for the ambulatory detoxification program include the following:

● Patient must have a DSM-IV diagnosis of substance-related disorder.
● Patient has a need for detoxification but is not at high risk for delirium tremens and other severe medical complications.
● Patient must be well enough to participate in the program.
● Patient requires an intensive day treatment program to complete detoxification safely.

The method of detoxification is 5 days a week, 6 hours per day, with daily medical status monitoring by a nurse and/or physician, open-ended groups with focused individual therapy, medication monitoring, random drug and alcohol screening, and a daily schedule that includes a combination of education and didactic therapy with medical monitoring and structured activities. The AA, NA, and Al-Anon philosophy is emphasized. Assessment by the nurse and/or medical director, monitoring of vital signs, administering medication, a lecture series, group therapy, a life skills group, a special focus therapy group, and individual treatment planning are formatted parts of the program, which runs from 10:00 A.M. to 5:00 P.M. Requirements include daily attendance, with absences reviewed by the counselor and medical director to determine continued participation or discharge. There must be a minimum attendance of three 12-Step meetings weekly. Each patient must keep a daily journal, complete assignments on time, accept random alcohol and drug screening, and comply with the medication regimen. The patient's medical condition must be stabilized before active participation.

Information discussed in the lectures includes the detoxification process, the disease of addiction, priorities, anger, family issues, physical problems, relapse prevention, support groups, feelings and regulation of affect, denial, powerlessness, grief and loss, cultural issues, adjusting to sobriety, responsibility, sexuality, communication, the genetics of addiction, the importance of focusing on oneself during the program, the symptoms of sobriety, change, and the first three steps of AA and NA. These are recurrent themes in the entire addiction program. Life skills training includes lifestyle awareness; setting priorities; determining values; using slogans; family teachings; sharing; practice; attitudes; self-honesty; decision making; reinforcing new actions; abstinence; dealing with people, places, and things; and choosing to change. Some types of focus groups include a men's group, a women's group, and focus groups that deal with responsibility, expression, learning to use AA, feelings, weekend plans, medication, powerlessness, self-honesty, sharing and fellowship, living with AIDS, self-worth, sexuality, and legal problems. The discharge criterion for the outpatient detoxification program is completion of the detoxification regimen. If the patient no longer meets the admission criteria, the patient may be referred to another level of care.

Partial Hospitalization

The trend from inpatient to outpatient and partial hospitalization programs has occurred because studies have found that outpatient and partial hospitalization programs enhance treatment effectiveness as much as inpatient programs and are more cost-effective. Clearly, some patients will need inpatient and rehabilitation programs. When necessary, patients are referred to longer-term inpatient psychiatric hospitals and residentially based programs. For the most part, however, our partial hospitalization program is able to provide a foundation for coping skills and behavioral and problem-solving techniques for our patients to achieve continuing sobriety and relapse prevention. The objectives of partial hospitalization are to learn techniques and develop skills to manage life's stresses within the work environment, family, and/or personal relationships; to recognize individual relapse triggers; and to learn to control them to prevent relapse. The program is geared to increase understanding of addictions and individual patterns of compulsive behavior that lead to relapse and to promote self-esteem, self-worth, and self-care to maintain sobriety.

Admission to the partial hospital program requires completion of an inpatient or outpatient detoxification program, with no medical or psychiatric complications requiring inpatient treatment. The patient should attend a daily, intensive, structured treatment program to promote recovery and would be at high risk for relapse without such a program. The method includes a 5-day-a-week, 6-hour-a-day, structured daily schedule, including a combination of cognitive-behavior therapy (lectures, life skills groups, focus groups), individual therapy weekly or as needed, family education, and medical monitoring as necessary. The daily schedule, which begins at 9:00 A.M. and ends at 4:00 P.M., includes a community meeting that reviews activities in the last 24 hours, a lecture series, group therapy, a life skills psychotherapy group, specially focused therapy groups, and individual therapy. The patient must attend a minimum of three 12-Step

meetings weekly, and each patient is required to keep a daily
journal, accept random alcohol and drug screenings, and comply with the medication regimen. The average length of stay in
the partial hospital program is 3–4 weeks. During the second
week, the patient is peer evaluated to help in assessment of motivation, to aid in confrontation of denial, and to add support.
The discharge criteria for partial hospitalization include that the
patient no longer meets the admission criteria and that the patient is referred to an appropriate level of care. The latter should
be decided by the team with the supervision of the director. The
patient should have completed the objectives of the individualized treatment plan, and the patient may be discharged if he or
she is noncompliant and abusing chemicals.

Intensive Outpatient Treatment Program

The organized outpatient program is 16 weeks' duration, with
opportunities for follow-up treatment. If Mr. M were to spend 1
week in an inpatient program, 4 weeks in an intensive partial
hospitalization program, 4 weeks in Phase I, and 6 weeks each
in Phase II and Phase III of the addiction treatment program, he
would have had a total of 21 weeks of treatment, after which he
would be placed in a follow-up program. After partial hospitalization, Mr. M could return to work or seek employment. Objectives for Phase I include increasing self-awareness and
understanding addiction, patterns of compulsive behavior, underlying issues, and the recovery process. Patients begin to develop skills that support independent thinking and behavior
based on sound problem-solving techniques and also learn to
set reasonable and realistic personal goals, develop a repertoire
of new interpersonal behavioral skills, and recognize and accept
patterns of cross-addiction and substitution as relapse triggers.
The 12-hour-a-week format (generally 3 hours a day) includes 9
hours of group therapy, 2 hours of individual therapy, and 1
hour of family therapy. Group membership is limited to a maxi-

mum of eight patients. Review of the treatment plan is required biweekly.

Requirements for Phase I include a commitment to attend at least four sessions within the first 4-week period and a minimum of three 12-Step meetings per week. It is also necessary to acquire a sponsor. Each individual who misses more than one group meeting is reviewed by the treatment team to determine continued participation. An individual who relapses is reviewed by the team for possible referral to another treatment level. The major focus is educational, with an effort at cognitive and behavioral approaches to teach methods for maintaining abstinence from mood-altering substances. The patient has the opportunity to learn how to live "one day at a time." Although 12-Step programs are strongly emphasized, some patients benefit from the professional treatment program without taking a self-help approach. Such patients are taught alternative coping and social skills to channel the energy of addictive-compulsive behavior and learn affect self-regulation. They learn to overcome shame, become edified from mistakes, and accept the responsibility and consequences for their behavior. Problem-solving and decision-making techniques as well as skills to recognize and express positive and negative feelings are emphasized. The program also uses relaxation techniques, explores rational versus irrational beliefs, and helps develop insight into self and addiction. Patients learn from the interpersonal interaction with the group, focus on acceptance of self, and learn to increase their tolerance for the problems of daily living. Individuals are helped to deal with anger, grief, loss, vulnerability, fear, and escape. The family, cultural impact, and realistic expectations are fostered. Patients discover how to recognize relapse triggers, their need to escape, and techniques for conflict resolution. These themes pervade treatment. Discharge criteria for Phase I include the patient no longer meets admission criteria, and the patient completes the objectives of the individualized treatment plan and is prepared for Phase II. Early discharge or transfer can occur with noncompliance.

Phase II is a 6-week program designed to strengthen personal growth for continuing recovery. The patient continues to expand and develop a repertoire of new interpersonal behavioral skills and increase the capacity for positive attitudes and behaviors to reinforce a chemically free lifestyle. The format is similar to Phase I. In Phase III, the focus is to transition the patient from the therapeutic situation to independent living successfully. This is accomplished with the assistance of support groups. Patients are required to attend sessions 3 days a week, a total of 9 hours, including 7 hours of group therapy, 1 hour of individual therapy, and 1 hour of family therapy. They also attend 12-Step meetings. Patients who relapse or regress during some aspect of the program are reevaluated by the team and referred to the appropriate level of care; however, the majority of patients proceed through the phases of treatment and maintain active recovery. Again, discharge depends on meeting objectives and readiness for Phase III.

The Alcohol Treatment Center has a family support program that helps family members understand the dynamics of compulsive behavior and learn the effects of substance abuse on the family, its emotional impact, and co-dependency issues. The objective of this program is to help family members increase self-awareness and skills to cope with the stress and frustration of living with or caring about someone with substance abuse problems. A weekly 1.5-hour group session for family members focuses on education and didactic methods. The impact on the family that compulsive behavior, co-dependency, replaying "family tapes," and repetition compulsion, as well as the emotions and feelings generated by having an addictive relative, have is an important part of the family's substance-abuse education. The average length of stay in the family program is 12 weeks.

The Addiction Treatment Center also has a 10-week, 1.5-hour weekly group program for adult children of alcoholics that helps patients build self-esteem and assertiveness and establish healthy personal relationships. In addition, the Addiction Treatment Center conducts an advanced women's recovery group for 1.5 hours weekly that addresses issues that women have in common as they seek sobriety. Women work on aspects of personal relationships; deal with neglect, abuse, and/or continued drinking by their spouse; and deal with issues of assertiveness, low self-esteem, guilt, shame, anxiety disorders, depression, and additional psychiatric problems. The focus is the prevention of relapse. The program is 12 weeks' duration on average and is limited to 12 members. Many women may have a need for a women's group that is a comfortable place to talk about sexual issues, physical and emotional abuse, problems in parenting, marital conflicts, and co-dependent behavior and may find great support from other members of the group, female friends, and female family members.

The Alcohol Treatment Center has a special program for intoxicated drivers that meets once a week for 1.5 hours over 16 sessions. It includes education, didactics, films, and discussion groups, with a special focus on maintaining recovery and instructing the patient about the danger of alcohol and drug use while driving. The program also helps patients accept the extent of their alcohol or drug problems. The Alcohol Treatment Center has an evening intensive outpatient program to meet the needs of patients who work in the community. The program, held five evenings per week, 4 hours per session, combines education and didactic, cognitive, and behavioral therapy with structured therapeutic activities. The program is scheduled from 5:30 P.M. until 10:00 P.M. and, to facilitate sobriety, includes a community meeting, a psychotherapy group, a specially focused group, a life skills group, and planned weekend discussions. In many ways, the educational program, with a length of stay of 4 weeks, parallels that of the organized outpatient treatment program.

Mentally Ill—Chemical Abuse Program

Mr. M can best be treated in the mentally ill—chemical abuse program as an alternative to the general program. This program attends to both his depression and chemical dependency because relapse in either illness can cause problems with both. This specialized track for patients with addictive disorders and mental illness helps patients achieve sobriety and accept the need for medication and other treatment for a psychiatric problem. In addition to the aims and objectives of our general adult track, the program increases understanding and acceptance of the addictive disorder, psychiatric disorder, patterns of compulsive behaviors, role of medication in the recovery process, and avoidance of iatrogenic dependency. Patients in this program must be age 18 years or older and have a diagnosis of substance-related disorder and a comorbid psychiatric disorder based on DSM-IV diagnosis.

The treatment program includes open therapeutic group sessions with cognitive-behavior psychotherapy (50%), addiction and mental health psychoeducation (20%), supportive therapy (20%), and evaluation of medications, side effects, and pharmacotherapy (10%). Patients receive individual cognitive-behavior psychotherapy for anxiety disorders, depression, and other psychiatric disorders, along with addiction treatment. Coping skills, stress reduction, and relapse prevention are important parts of the treatment program. For women, there is a special focus on dual diagnosis and network support when marital problems interfere. The format is a 1.5-hour therapeutic group, four times per week, with 1 hour of therapy weekly and network and family evaluation and treatment when indicated. Group therapy is required four times a week and individual, family, or network therapy once a week, as specified in the individual treatment plan. Patients must attend at least two AA, NA, or dual-diagnosis support meetings per week and have a sponsor. The average length of stay is approximately 24 weeks, but the duration is tailored to one's needs. Treatment plans are individualized, and managing psychiatric symptoms is synchronized with the recovery process for addiction.

Adolescent Drug and Alcohol Prevention and Treatment Unit

The Adolescent Drug and Alcohol Prevention Treatment program has similar goals as the adult program, with special emphasis on improving self-esteem, coping, and problem-solving skills to manage personal growth and development, free of all mood- and mind-altering drugs and alcohol. The objectives are also similar in that special emphasis is placed on family and peer relationships with methods specific to adolescent development. The development of appropriate interpersonal relationships, an understanding of the disease concept of addiction, and working through some of the special resistances to treatment that are likely to occur with adolescents are integral components of the program, which relies heavily on peer group input, support, and role-modeling.

Admission criteria include the primary diagnosis of a substance-related disorder that meets the DSM-IV diagnostic criteria. Participants are between the ages of 12 and 20 years old. A biopsychosocial evaluation comparable to that used in the adult program is completed, but it contains a treatment agreement that must be signed by the adolescent pledging that he or she will be self-motivated. Treatment methods include cognitive-behavior therapy (50%), peer support therapy (20%), addiction psychoeducation (15%), and adolescent development psychoeducation (15%). Individual psychotherapy, family therapy as needed, and participation in organized social recreational activities that serve as an alternative to chemical use are also encouraged.

The program is 4 hours per week, comprising two 1.5-hour group therapy sessions and a 1-hour individual therapy session. An additional hour may be required each week for family therapy. Participation in self-help groups is also recommended. The educational focus is similar to that of the adult program, with an emphasis on developmental issues of adolescents, including problems with authority, socialization, self-responsibility, self-care, self-esteem, body image, and alternatives to chemical use (e.g., exercise, sports, and positive social involvement). The program is organized in three phases, with increasing involvement of the family. Each phase focuses on specific objectives, and treatment is tailored to the patient's individual needs. Completion of the program takes 25 weeks; the average length of stay is 20 weeks.

Conclusion

A full range of programs constituting the alcohol and addiction service line at Hackensack University Medical Center has been described. Some of the programs have only recently commenced operation, and someday we hope to have treatment outcome data on all programs. Clearly, aspects of the programs will change with shifts in the patient population, outcome research literature, and economics of care delivery. Our staff has learned to be flexible, to incorporate new techniques, and to update their clinical skills constantly. Staff development and education are crucial to ensure optimal care. Our efforts aim to tailor appropriate treatment for patients such as Mr. M, who are offered greater hope for recovery when a range of quality services is available.

Reference

American Psychiatric Association: Diagnostic and Statistical Manual of Mental Disorders, 4th Edition. Washington, DC, American Psychiatric Association, 1994

Additional Readings

Frances RJ, Franklin JE: A Concise Guide to Treatment of Alcoholism and Addictions. Washington, DC, American Psychiatric Press, 1989
Frances RJ, Miller SI: Clinical Textbook of Addictive Disorders. New York, Guilford, 1991
Horgan C: Substance Abuse: The Nation's Number One Health Problem: Key Indications for Policy. Princeton, New Jersey, Institute for Health Policy, Brandeis University for the Robert Wood Johnson Foundation, October 1993

8 Acute Inpatient Treatment

Robert Wisner-Carlson, M.D.

Managed care is the latest in a long line of assailants to the inpatient ward. Twenty years ago, Maxmen et al. (1974), in their book *Rational Hospital Psychiatry: The Reactive Environment,* attempted to show how the psychiatric hospital "still has an important place in the care of many emotionally disturbed individuals" (p. 20). They defined *short term* as an average length of stay of less than 3 weeks. Now hospital stays are defined in days, and many psychiatrists are wondering what they can accomplish therapeutically in so short a time.

The Short-Term Treatment Unit at Sheppard Pratt Hospital opened September 1992 to meet the demand by managed care companies and health maintenance organizations for a brief crisis stabilization approach to inpatient treatment. The unit has treated more than 2,000 patients in its 3 years of operation, achieving an average length of stay of 6 days. Half the patients are discharged in 5 or fewer days. This is accomplished by rapidly gathering pertinent information to make a diagnosis, setting limited treatment goals aimed at stabilizing the patient's crisis, and then referring the patient to an appropriate lower level of care. All the major diagnoses are treated on the unit, with the top three diagnoses being major depression, bipolar disorder, and adjustment disorder(s). The screening criterion for admission to the unit is that a patient is dangerous, either to him- or herself or to others, or possesses a degree of disorganization that is potentially dangerous. At least two-thirds of the patients are suicidal. They are referred from the entire continuum, but always after a screening assessment. Thus, patients are referred from emergency rooms, mobile crisis programs, day programs, clinics, and therapists' offices. The staffing needed to accomplish this is described in Table 8–1.

Suicidal patients are evaluated with three goals in mind: 1) to determine the patient's degree of dangerousness, 2) to make a diagnosis, and 3) to pinpoint the key problems to be addressed during the hospitalization. Thus, how dangerous is the individual and what is causing the danger? These questions are answered through interviewing and observing the patient and gathering collateral information from family, friends, and sometimes co-workers. We want to gather the most information in the least amount of time possible.

The psychiatrist calls the outpatient providers (e.g., psychiatrist, therapist, internist, gynecologist, primary care physician). The outpatient diagnosis and history may illuminate the reasons for this crisis admission. The social worker contacts the family and/or significant others to obtain their observations and descriptions of problems occurring in this crisis. The psychiatrist and social worker make their contacts within the first 24 hours of the admission. Patients with bipolar disorder (including mixed states), psychosis, substance abuse, and personality disorders can all present with depression and suicidal ideation.

Table 8–1.	Staff composition and staff-to-patient ratios
Discipline	**Staff:patient**
Psychiatry	1:9
Nursing	1:5
Social work	1:5

Making the proper diagnosis guides the treatment and often depends on obtaining good collateral history.

The dangerousness assessment involves understanding the lethality of the suicide attempt. Was the person intending to kill him- or herself and is the person still suicidal? The treatment team seeks to put together a clear picture of the suicide attempt and the events leading up to it. What was the patient doing before the overdose? How long had the patient been considering suicide? What plans had been made to complete the suicide? Did the patient leave a suicide note? Was the person intoxicated during the suicide attempt? Did the patient get drunk to kill him- or herself or did the patient become suicidal after becoming drunk? Was the overdose impulsive after an argument or was it planned over several weeks? Numerous articles review the assessment of suicide and are applicable to this setting (Brent et al. 1988).

Suicidal patients often feel disconnected from their support system. This alienation may arise from their family's lack of understanding of a major depression. There may be a marital or family conflict that needs to be resolved. The crisis may relate to a work issue. An employee assistance program counselor may be helpful in this regard.

> Mrs. B is a 38-year-old woman admitted after a pill overdose with continued suicidality. She has no past psychiatric history. She has been suffering from major depressive symptoms over the last 6–8 weeks. She has never drunk heavily, but in the last 2 weeks she has begun to drink at least half a bottle of wine at night to put herself to sleep. She has felt worthless and has had thoughts of death for about a week before the pill overdose. The day of the overdose, the patient had gone to work, and her supervisor met with her to tell her of her poor work performance lately. That evening, she got into an argument with her husband over her increased drinking and her inattention to household chores. He called her an alcoholic and threatened to walk out on her. He left the house, and Mrs. B took an overdose of acetaminophen and about half a bottle of wine. She did not leave a suicide note. About 2 hours later, Mrs. B called her

sister and told her what she had done, and the sister called 911.

In Mrs. B's case, the psychiatrist's diagnosis was major depression, single episode, and alcohol abuse. The social worker educated the husband about the patient's illness ("depressed, not lazy") on the second hospital day. Antidepressant medication was begun. The patient denied suicidal ideation and felt more hopeful that she was being heard by her family. She felt more connected. She agreed to have her employee assistance program counselor contacted by the social worker. The employee assistance program counselor at her workplace indicated that with Mrs. B's permission, feedback about her depression would be provided to her boss.

Mrs. B was discharged on the third hospital day with immediate follow-up in the day program. There, her vital signs would continue to be monitored for alcohol withdrawal. Outpatient psychiatric and individual therapy appointments were arranged for the day after (while she was still attending the day program). The outpatient therapist was given clinical information, including information about the patient's alcohol abuse. He would follow up on this problem in outpatient therapy.

In this case, the patient clearly had a major depression that was fueling the suicidal ideation. However, the depression was causing problems in several spheres of her life. The final straw was the disconnection the patient felt from her family. Although the patient was demoralized and hopeless, the hopelessness did not grow directly out of the depression but rather out of the effects of the depression on her life. After the suicide attempt, the family, and to some extent her boss, could be educated about her depressive illness. These interventions remoralized the patient. Although she continued to feel depressed, she was no longer hopeless and disconnected. The suicidal ideation thus waned.

Demoralization and remoralization are important phenomena on the acute inpatient ward. In their classic book, *Persua-*

sion and Healing: A Comparative Study of Psychotherapy, Frank and Frank (1991) described these phenomena in outpatient psychotherapy and believed remoralization to be one of the therapeutic actions of all psychotherapies. Beck et al. (1975, 1985) wrote about the role of hopelessness in depression and suicide. The depressed, suicidal patient on the crisis ward is usually hopeless and demoralized. Action and structure of the ward are organized with the goal of reversing this demoralization and hopelessness.

The hospitalization and the rituals surrounding admission are remoralizing for many patients. The patient's problems have reached a critical point and are made known to family and significant others. There is a promise that the problems will be resolved. Barriers to communication are broken down; what was hidden is now disclosed. Energies for change are mobilized. A patient can reach out to his or her family, friends, and co-workers, who—now knowledgeable of the situation—can support the patient.

However, problems and issues between the patient and the patient's support system can interfere with this remoralization process. Sometimes, simply educating family, friends, and perhaps co-workers about the patient's mental illness helps. At other times, there are specific conflicts between the patient and these individuals. The social worker attempts to work out these conflicts so that the support system can be supportive to the patient once again, but this may not be possible. For example, sometimes a crisis has flared because a couple is ready to separate or divorce. Discussing this and coming to some resolution about this may be the therapeutic activity of the hospitalization.

Mrs. B's suicidality was due to a circumscribed set of problems that could be quickly and efficiently dealt with. Another example is the patient who becomes suicidal only when intoxicated. Although many of these individuals are stabilized in an emergency room, many are admitted to an inpatient ward for treatment.

> Mr. F is a 32-year-old married man with a 10-year history of alcohol and crack cocaine use. He was admitted because he

tried to hang himself while intoxicated on these substances. Collateral history from his wife revealed escalating suicidal statements by the patient over the last month, including threatening to shoot himself with his revolver. These statements always occurred when the patient was intoxicated. On admission to the ward, the patient was denying suicidal ideation. He admitted that he had made suicidal statements on a number of occasions while intoxicated.

The patient was admitted on a Saturday evening. The weekend social worker met with the patient and his wife on the second hospital day, a Sunday afternoon. His wife expressed her thorough disgust with his substance abuse and threatened to leave him. She relented when he promised to enter intensive substance abuse treatment. The social worker also discussed the issue of the gun. The patient agreed that his wife should give the gun to her brother, who would keep it double-locked in his home. On the third hospital day, the patient's mood was improving. He had no suicidal ideation. He was showing no signs of alcohol withdrawal. Because the patient's substance abuse was escalating for a month before admission and now was having immediate life-threatening consequences, arrangements were made for the patient's transfer to a residential substance abuse program. There he would receive intensive substance abuse treatment in a moderately monitored setting. He could continue to be monitored for suicidal ideation and hopelessness in this setting, as well as for signs and symptoms of alcohol withdrawal. After an expected residential stay of about 2 weeks, he would be transferred to a lower level of care. He and his wife were satisfied with the transfer to the residential substance abuse program, which occurred on the third hospital day.

Unique aspects of staffing allowed for the rapid treatment and transfer of Mr. F. Coverage by social workers is 7 days per week and about 10 hours per day on weekdays. This coverage allows for rapid collection of collateral information. Social workers also are available to meet with families immediately after admission.

Another important part of the staffing is integrating the utilization review nurse into the treatment team. The nurse attends all the team meetings and interacts directly with the managed care company. This interaction helps clarify insurance benefits and treatment options. In this example, the patient's insurance covered residential substance abuse treatment. The lack of this benefit or the lack of knowledge about it would have unnecessarily prolonged the patient's hospital stay.

Some patients threatening suicide are not really suicidal. These include patients who, although self-destructive, are making suicidal statements to manipulate interpersonal interactions. Some patients are not patients at all and simply want to get out of some "tight place." The former must be distinguished from the latter. The patient who recurrently expresses distress through statements of self-harm needs assistance in dealing with these problems. The latter, masquerading as a patient, needs to be found out and, if appropriate, turned over to the authorities. Both situations are facilitated by good collateral information gathering.

In the examples of Mrs. B and Mr. F, depression and alcohol abuse, respectively, caused unraveling of their lives, leading to hopelessness and suicidal behavior. For other patients, dangerousness is more closely linked to the symptoms of the psychiatric condition. The severely depressed patient may have feelings of extreme guilt, worthlessness, helplessness, and hopelessness as symptoms of the depression. Only suicide makes sense to this patient. Or the patient may have delusional beliefs or auditory hallucinations "demanding" suicide of him or her. Patients with schizophrenia or mania may be too agitated or disorganized to be safe out of a 24-hour monitored setting. When symptoms are severe and dangerousness grows directly out of the psychiatric condition, more thorough treatment is needed to allow discharge. Intermediate levels of care, including short-term therapeutic living situations coupled with day programs, can shorten hospital stays by acting as "step-down" services.

Mr. D is a 33-year-old single man admitted involuntarily with religious delusions, auditory hallucinations, irritabil-

Managing Care, Not Dollars

ity, labile mood, and violent behavior. His history was significant for psychiatric problems intermittently for more
than 10 years, with regular return to his premorbid level of
functioning. The patient had been regularly employed until
this psychotic episode, which may have been precipitated
by substance abuse.

During the hospitalization, the patient initially would
not take medication. After 2 days, his family was able to convince him to start medications. He became even more compliant with medications after he was retained at an
involuntary commitment hearing. He made sufficient improvement to be discharged on the ninth hospital day. He
was sleeping at night and was not physically agitated or verbally threatening. His mood was much less labile. However,
he continued to have delusions and to experience some
auditory hallucinations. He was not insightful about his
condition, and he gave the impression he would not comply with his medications. Thus, he was transferred directly
to a 24-hour acute residential setting, in addition to attending a day program, where he would stay for an additional
10 days. He was willing to take an injection of depot
neuroleptic before discharge from the inpatient setting.

When patients are admitted with an acute psychotic disorder
(with hallucinations, delusions, and disordered thoughts), disorganized and agitated, stabilization must occur within a 24-
hour highly monitored setting. The patient may continue to be
psychotic, disorganized, and somewhat agitated for some time
(a few days to a couple of weeks), and it may be inappropriate
for the patient to be left alone at home or under the care of the
family. In this situation, day programs, short-term residential
programs, home psychiatric nursing, and crisis intervention
teams can be helpful in allowing discharge from the inpatient
setting while continuing to provide a high level of care.

The average length of stay for patients with bipolar disorder
(manic) or schizophrenia is more in the range of 8–10 days, although such patients may stay a couple to several weeks and
rarely a month or two. However, even with such long lengths of

stay, we have been able to keep the average length of stay to about 6 days, with a median of 5 days. Thus, resources are shifted to those patients who are particularly vulnerable and require constant nursing observation and assessment to stay safe.

Not all patients who are admitted with mania or schizophrenia are hallucinating and delusional. Psychosocial problems also, of course, affect this group of patients and do so without causing a full relapse in the illness. The application of our psychosocial treatment to these situations can often resolve them sufficiently to allow treatment to continue out of the hospital.

Special Challenges and Problems With This Level of Care

The brief-stay crisis stabilization ward presents unique challenges for all involved in its operation: ward staff, patients and families, and referrers.

Staff

Crisis stabilization is high-intensity work. Some individuals walking through the ward have compared it to an emergency room. Thus, the potential for staff burnout and rapid turnover is high. Compared with staff in less acute settings, the staff in the crisis stabilization ward has less ability to develop extended relationships with the patient. One staff member, only partly in jest, said, "When patients are well enough to really discuss things, they're discharged."

Patients in crisis are distraught and disorganized. They are often coarse in their interpersonal interactions. The hues and nuances of their personalities and their sense of humor are temporarily lost. Indeed, as soon as these start to return, the individual is usually doing well enough to be discharged. This phenomenon is difficult for staff who are in this profession specifically because they value and enjoy the professional relationships they have with people who are experiencing psychiatric troubles.

Therefore, the right temperament in the staff is extremely important on such a ward. One needs staff with experience and perspective. Because many psychiatric conditions last for months or years, staff need perspective on how this crisis and inpatient admission fit into the scheme of the patient's ongoing illness. However, staff need to thrive on the fast-paced activity and decision making necessary for such a brief admission. They need to enjoy the rapid, albeit sometimes incomplete, changes an individual can make during a crisis stabilization admission.

The short-term stay works because of the alternatives to inpatient care that are available (e.g., intensive outpatient treatment, day programs, in-home treatment, temporary therapeutic living situations). Someone on the team needs to know these alternative levels of care, how to access them, and their functional reality; that is, will this alternative level of care really address the patient's and family's needs in all practical reality?

The shorter length of stay also can wreak havoc on the census. This is because admissions come in waves with crests and troughs, not in a steady stream. To make the unit run financially efficiently, one must be able to bring in and release staff fluidly. This issue causes problems. The ward operates on a team model, and members of the team must develop sufficient rapport to work well together; this takes time. One must strike a balance between staffing continuity and financial constraints. Having individuals who work part-time and who are willing to increase hours, individuals who work regularly on the ward on an occasional basis, individuals who work in a float pool, and a high-quality reliable staffing agency can be helpful. Of course, when the census goes down, staff sometimes just need a break from the work.

Patients and Family

Most of the difficulty for patients and their families with short-term hospitalization centers around their expectations. Some patients and families expect more: more psychotherapy time, more family time with the psychiatrist, and more improvement before discharge. Patients, and their families, sometimes expect they will be well before discharge (e.g., normal mood—not depressed, not hearing voices, not delusional). These disagreements in the ultimate goal of the hospitalization impair both patient satisfactionand remoralization. Educating the patient and family at the outset about treatment philosophy and average length of stay for the unit can make expectations more realistic.

Other patients show more of a dependency on the hospital. One must be aware of this potential in a given patient and help move the situation along before dependency sets in and regression occurs. Sometimes this means judging whether the patient's statements about being safe in the hospital but not out of the hospital are an honest expression of a careful self-assessment or an expression of the patient's dependency on the hospital. Because of the difficulty in predicting dangerous behaviors (suicide), the clinician's opinion and subjective judgment play a large role in determining when the patient can be (and sometimes should be) discharged.

The activities of the ward are structured to reduce dependency and to encourage self-motivation and forward movement. Patients are expected to attend all appropriate groups and activities. Patients are not allowed to isolate themselves in their rooms. Discharge planning begins at the moment of admission, and patients have to face the fact of discharge immediately.

Referrers

Referrers' expectations for the hospitalization may differ depending on their outpatient mode of practice. Those referrers who are familiar with alternative levels of care and have the resources to deal with very ill patients on an outpatient basis will have no trouble with short-term hospitalization. However, other outpatient referrers may not be as flexible and receptive of the crisis intervention model. This can cause difficulty in arranging timely outpatient or day patient appointments. Even more difficult is when the outpatient provider has different goals for the hospitalization than the inpatient treatment team. These situations need to be carefully negotiated, and the outpatient provider needs to be informed about the goals of brief-stay crisis stabilization.

Summary

Although hospital admission rates and lengths of stay have dramatically fallen, the inpatient psychiatric ward continues to have an important role in the treatment of psychiatric conditions. The reason for hospitalization is crisis stabilization of a dangerous situation. This crisis is usually suicide but also includes disorganization (usually due to psychosis) and dangerous behavior toward others. Crisis stabilization is effectively provided by performing efficient and focused treatment. The program needs to operate 7 days per week, including weekend staffing of social workers and physicians. With the right staffing and treatment philosophy, expedient assessments will lead to immediate treatment interventions. The crisis stabilization ward provides challenges for staff, patients, families, and referral sources. Timely education of all parties involved helps to avoid conflicts.

References

Beck AT, Kovacs M, Weissman A: Hopelessness and suicidal behavior: an overview. JAMA 234:1146–1149, 1975
Beck AT, Steer RA, Kovacs M, et al: Hopelessness and eventual suicide: a 10-year prospective study of patients hospitalized with suicidal ideation. Am J Psychiatry 142:559–563, 1985
Brent DA, Kupfer DJ, Bromet EJ, et al: The assessment and treatment of patients at risk for suicide, in American Psychiatric Press Review of Psychiatry, Vol 7. Edited by Frances AJ, Hales RE. Washington, DC, American Psychiatric Press, 1988, pp 353–385

Frank JD, Frank JB: Persuasion and Healing: A Comparative Study of Psychotherapy, 3rd Edition. Baltimore, MD, Johns Hopkins University Press, 1991

Maxmen JS, Tucker GJ, LeBow MD: Rational Hospital Psychiatry: The Reactive Environment. New York, Brunner/Mazel, 1974

Additional Readings

Frank JD, Frank JB: A conceptual framework for psychotherapy, in Persuasion and Healing: A Comparative Study of Psychotherapy, 3rd Edition. Baltimore, MD, Johns Hopkins University Press, 1991, pp 21–51

Kennedy P, Hird F: Description and evaluation of a short-stay admission ward. Br J Psychiatry 136:205–215, 1980

Weisman G, Feirstein A, Thomas C: Three-day hospitalization—a model for intensive intervention. Arch Gen Psychiatry 12:620–629, 1969

II

Using the Continuum
for Children,
Adolescents, and
the Elderly

9 Foster Care

Alvin A. Rosenfeld, M.D.
Richard Altman, M.S.W.
Ira Kaufman, M.S.W.

Managed care companies have incorporated a wide spectrum of mental health services, searching for economical ways to provide a seamless continuum of patient care. Although the efforts have included traditional Joint Commission on Accreditation of Healthcare Organizations–approved mental health settings, to date, managed care companies' primary interest in foster care has been getting that system's assistance in transferring children and adolescents from private to public facilities.

The foster care system is usually thought of as a child welfare system with family boarding homes. In fact, it has evolved into a broad spectrum of services, including residential treatment facilities, step-down facilities, diagnostic centers, day hospitals, group homes, boarding homes, therapeutic foster homes, regular foster homes, and preventive services.

In this chapter, we briefly review foster care's history, giving perspective on its current status. Using primarily our experience at the Jewish Child Care Association, which was founded in 1822 and now serves children regardless of their ethnic, religious, or racial backgrounds, we describe the scope of contemporary foster care, the populations this system serves, and the services it delivers. Many foster care services we list are discussed elsewhere in this book, in Chapters 10 through 12. In this chapter, we focus on an extension of current foster boarding home services in which managed care companies have expressed great interest, a proposed therapeutic foster family program that could be a new, useful component in a seamless, comprehensive spectrum of services for children and adolescents.

History

Foster care's origins reach back to the first human beings who had to decide what to do with orphans or with children whose parents were unwilling or unable to care for them. By the mid-20th century, public hygiene had improved, malnutrition had become far less prevalent, medications were available to treat diseases such as tuberculosis and syphilis, and financial supports were available to indigent parents. Illnesses that had left children parentless, temporarily or permanently, no longer were a scourge. Foster family homes began serving an increasing number of children who were (or who had parents who were) emotionally disturbed. Child welfare institutions—orphanages in particular—shifted their mission and became parts of large foster care agencies. In the 1960s and 1970s, they transformed themselves into residential treatment centers for children and adolescents; many of these children were seriously disturbed psychiatrically. Residential treatment centers that some religious groups built for co-religionists became secularized (for a more complete history, see Rosenfeld et al. 1994).

As public funding began to pay for many indigent, emotionally disturbed youngsters, private philanthropy diminished. States "deinstitutionalized" mental health services for children. That shifted responsibility for many seriously disturbed children from specialized medical providers, such as state-run psychiatric hospitals, to more generic foster care services in the child welfare system. Local authorities who needed to place psychiatrically disturbed youngsters were glad to refer them to less costly foster care residential treatment facilities. The private nonprofit agency facilities and the state funding became intertwined and mutually interdependent.

From the 1970s to the present, disturbed and disturbing children were placed in ever less restrictive environments. Foster care's institutions served increasingly more severely ill children. Those who traditionally had been placed in residential facilities were sent to less restrictive group homes and foster homes. Children who previously would have been in psychiatric hospitals now went to residential facilities, perhaps after a brief hospital stay. In the 20 years since this process took hold, the better residential treatment centers, group homes, and youth residences in the foster care system have acquired substantial expertise in dealing with severely mentally ill children and adolescents in nonhospital settings. To do so, they hired more psychiatrists, psychologists, and social workers. They developed quiet rooms, infirmaries, and diagnostic units. Over those two decades, children referred to and accepted for care had increasingly more severe psychiatric histories and needs. For example, at the Pleasantville Cottage School (a Jewish Child Care Association 200-bed residential facility in Westchester County, New York, that once had been a Jewish orphan asylum), approximately 50% of the residents (most of whom come from minority groups) have been hospitalized psychiatrically. Despite the treatment center's efforts to take children off psychotropic medications, as many as 50% of them continue to need them. These percentages are lower in less restrictive settings such as group homes and family foster homes.

Despite the high level of services, public funding sources have exerted strong, at times unrealistic, pressure on the agencies to contain costs. Therefore, even though these facilities deal effectively with all but the most disturbed and disturbing children, current staffing levels and costs per day remain substantially below those in mental health facilities.

In recent years, however, the relationship between private not-for-profit agencies and public funders has become more strained, at times near the breaking point. At the same time, managed care companies and hospitals have been looking for well-run, cost-effective services to collaborate with. In many states, Medicaid, which helps fund many foster care facilities, has been moving toward a managed care model. This has led to increasingly frequent conversations, and at times collaborations, among facilities in the foster care system, managed care companies, and hospitals organizing comprehensive systems of care.

Services

The current foster care system provides a full spectrum of mental health services. In this section, we briefly describe these services, from the least to the most restrictive. Then, a newly proposed therapeutic foster home program is described in greater detail.

Foster Care Options: Child Welfare Service Provision

Foster homes.   Foster family homes are the least restrictive primary placement for infants and preschool-age children who need to live with other families. Latency-age children and adolescents can also benefit from these homes if their behavior is not too disruptive and their needs not too extreme. The foster family is supported by a social work case manager; psychiatric and psychological services often are minimal, usually being available on a crisis basis. The foster family home, combined with psychotherapy, is supposed to be sufficient to alter the children's disturbed emotional and psychiatric state. Children who rebel against living in a substitute family, those who are overtly dangerous to themselves and others, and those with extremely fragile ego development or seriously underdeveloped impulse control need more than a foster home can provide: a more structured setting that includes regular, on-site professional support and intervention. Older adolescent males may have difficulty being served in this system.

Foster care agencies in many localities, and private firms in others, find and supervise foster families. They have developed expertise in selecting families who will be warm and nurturing and who will support the child's healthy growth. The foster care agency is also responsible for monitoring the placement with the foster family and with trying to reunite the child with the biological family as soon as possible. Where this clearly is impossible, the agency seeks adoptive parents to assume permanent responsibility for the child. Because not all seriously troubled children can benefit from regular foster care, many localities have developed therapeutic foster home programs.

Therapeutic foster homes.   In an effort to provide more intensive services, or to shorten hospital and residential treatment center stays, many localities have developed more professional, more highly trained foster families who could care for seriously disturbed children and adolescents.

"Regular" foster care has operated on the idea that good-enough parents in a good-enough home can, with only a modest amount of training and supervision, be an adequate placement for most children needing out-of-home care. Therapeutic foster care is the foster care system's best effort to date to develop a "professional foster parent" with respect for the position, a clear role, and tasks as a full professional team member. These parents get far more training, ongoing supervision, respite care, and readily available professional input. Therapeutic foster homes, which Fine (1993) called "residential therapy within a family setting," provide children and adolescents with an in-home treatment environment that helps them develop adequate competence to function in the everyday world, a better sense of themselves, and higher self-esteem. Therapeutic foster homes use the relationship with the foster family as a therapeutic tool, a model relationship that promotes development and within which helpful, corrective, and/or compensatory social and emotional experiences can occur for both the children and their birth parents.

Foster families who take on the responsibilities of therapeutic foster parenting need more than a wholesome family life and good parenting skills. These families must accept the fact that the child coming into their home has serious mental health problems that require attention and special intervention methods. They must be selected carefully. These foster parents are trained more intensively, paid higher stipends, and function as part of an interdisciplinary team of psychiatrists, psychologists, social workers, nurses, educators, and child care workers.

In addition to the family living (which serves as a day-to-day milieu approach), the therapeutic foster home program provides psychotherapy, psychopharmacology, crisis management, targeted family intervention, and special educational services as part of the care plan. Simultaneously, the staff and foster parents work with the biological families to remediate interactive styles that have made it difficult for the children and their birth and/or extended families to live together. When the children are well enough, they should be ready to return to their birth families or to go to a "regular" foster home with less intensive services. This relatively new form of care will require evaluation and outcome studies to determine its efficacy.

Below, we propose a new model of therapeutic foster care applicable to the managed care world.

Group homes.   When the special needs of children and adolescents with behavioral disorders and emotional disturbances exceed a therapeutic foster family's ability, a foster care boarding or group home can be a viable, valuable, and cost-effective option. The child welfare system currently operates numerous group homes that can fill this role. Specifics of group homes are discussed by Stone (Chapter 10, in this volume).

Day treatment services.   Many foster care agencies operate day treatment programs for children and adolescents. Like day treatment facilities in the mental health system, foster care day treatment programs remedy learning deficiencies, ameliorate depression and alienation, and help shape and improve academic, vocational, and social competencies. By providing therapeutic management 5 days per week, as well as weekend backup for psychiatric emergencies, day treatment programs affiliated with comprehensive foster care programs often are valuable resources that managed care providers can use for children and adolescents with serious psychological, behavioral, psychiatric, or social needs. Specifics about these programs are discussed by Stone (Chapter 10, in this volume).

Diagnostic centers. Residential treatment center–based diagnostic centers perform multidisciplinary comprehensive assessments of children and adolescents and are used for crisis management when, because of issues of safety and security, patients must be removed from their families. In cases where placement cannot be avoided, the diagnostic center is often the locus from which planning for placement in a foster home, group home, or residential treatment center can occur. In most situations, excellent centers can do thorough evaluations and make recommendations at costs substantially below hospital rates.

Residential treatment centers. Today, children are sent to both the foster care system's and the private sector's residential treatment centers only when their needs cannot be provided for in other less restrictive facilities. Primary in the assessment for this level of care is this key question: What specific interventions are required to help this patient that are not available in the community? Because these foster care residential centers have a relatively high staffing ratio, they can care for all but the most severely and acutely psychiatrically ill patients, at costs far more modest than those of hospitals and private-sector residential facilities. For instance, children and adolescents whose behavior or psychological disturbance constitutes a danger to themselves or others often can be served at a residential treatment center without ever being hospitalized. Residential treatment centers also can be used as step-down transitional settings after short-term psychiatric hospitalization for acute, severe psychiatric situations or as an alternative to hospitalization. These facilities are discussed in depth by Stone (Chapter 10, in this volume).

Therapeutic Foster Home Services: A Proposal for a New Service

Current service systems hope that specially trained and supervised foster homes can be viable therapeutic alternatives to prolonged hospitalizations and residential center stays. We propose a therapeutic foster home model that could serve children and adolescents manifesting significant psychopathology and behavioral difficulties. It is constructed from what we know about foster care as well as from what we know from our experience with more intensive levels of care. This service might fill a void in the current spectrum of managed care mental health services.

The model we propose utilizes an interdisciplinary treatment team working collaboratively with intensively trained therapeutic foster families to achieve clearly defined treatment outcomes. This therapeutic foster home model provides a milieu that helps troubled children and adolescents overcome their difficulties while they become more competent living in the day-to-day world. Simultaneously, both staff and foster parents work with biological parents to facilitate the child's return home, whenever this is possible, or to his or her transition to a less intensively staffed foster home or adoption.

All patients selected for referral to a therapeutic foster home would have at least a DSM-IV (American Psychiatric Association 1994) diagnosis on Axis I. Symptomatology must be stable and manageable within a foster home in the community.

Patient population.   Patients must be selected carefully for a therapeutic foster home. Four broad categories of patients should be considered:

1. *Children and adolescents who have been hospitalized psychiatrically and cannot return to their own families be-*

cause parenting resources are inadequate or because severe conflicts make the patients and their families unable to live together at this time. These patients often remain in hospitals for long periods of time or go home only to be rehospitalized shortly after discharge. A successful transfer to a therapeutic foster home milieu could spare great expense and equally great emotional damage from regression in their clinical condition.

2. *Children and adolescents who need psychiatric hospitalization for an acute psychotic episode but whose home situation cannot support them on discharge.* The hospital stays for these patients could be shortened if they were placed in an intensive therapeutic foster home.

3. *Children and adolescents who are chronically ill psychiatrically.* These patients often remain in psychiatric hospitals with no defined discharge goals, and they need safety, care, and support. Many could be served, and served better, in therapeutic foster homes.

4. *Children and adolescents who suffer from chronic, "psychologically related" physical illness, such as asthma, diabetes, or anorexia nervosa.* These patients often do very well with only brief hospital stays. Soon after they return to their biological families, they deteriorate. For these patients, 10 medical hospitalizations within a 2-year period are not unheard of. Therapeutic foster home placement is a viable alternative to the debilitating "yo-yo" experience these patients have and would help prevent a good part of the expenditures of repeated medical hospitalization.

A skilled clinical team is utilized to separate out inappropriate referrals. *Severely aggressive or overtly violent patients, predatory sexual offenders, and most fire setters would be inappropriate.*

Therapeutic foster parents. The recruitment, selection, training, supervision, and ongoing support of the therapeutic foster parents are the centerpiece of developing a successful program.

Because the foster parents are the primary therapeutic agents and because they function with a large degree of autonomy day to day, they must be aggressively supported in their effort to deliver high-quality therapeutic services.

Recruitment campaigns ought to include advertisements in newspapers, radio and television announcements, fliers, word of mouth, and so on. All advertisements ought to focus on attracting a large pool of potential foster families willing and interested enough to make a telephone inquiry. All callers are invited to a general inquirers' meeting where they are told about the program's goals and philosophy, the patients to be served, and the scope and nature of the training for foster parents. Videotapes are shown that bring the information to life and help inquirers decide whether this demanding venture really appeals to them. At the end of this meeting, all those who continue to express an interest are given an application. Because people need time to think through making a major commitment, potential applicants are encouraged to wait at least 24 hours before deciding whether to return the application.

The family is then asked to attend two precertification group meetings. This gives the whole therapeutic team a chance to meet and interact with the applicants. If they still are interested, and if the staff considers them suitable, the family is assigned to a member of the program's professional team. A formal home study is initiated. The home study must be careful, thorough, and intense. It is a wide-ranging interview designed to elicit information about the family's level of concern for children, child-rearing beliefs and practices, attitudes about discipline and structure, economic stability, and ability to function as a member of a larger service team.

The home study also assesses the family's frustration tolerance level, creativity, resourcefulness, nuclear and extended family relationships, natural children's adjustment and feelings about foster children being placed in their home, relationship to and attitude about the educational system, community affiliations and memberships, religious practices and beliefs, leisure time activities, attitudes and feelings about work, and ability to interact and attitudes about interacting with biological families of placed foster children. It includes a visit to the home to inspect the physical site and ensure that the prospective therapeutic foster family maintains acceptable standards of cleanliness, space, ventilation, safety, and privacy. The home study normally takes two to three separate interviews and includes all members of the household. If the program is to function well, deficiencies and problems within the home must be uncovered, just as strengths and attributes need to be discovered and highlighted.

In addition, in New York, applicants must submit their names to the New York State child abuse registry to determine whether they have a prior record of abuse or neglect. They also must provide personal and business references and undergo medical examinations. Some localities fingerprint applicants, eliminating those with a criminal record. The professional service team reviews the home study. If they approve the home, the family is certified as a therapeutic foster home and is assigned for intensive training. In general, good foster families are hard to find. We have been pleasantly surprised, however, to find that among those deemed suitable, many foster parents are very willing to take on great therapeutic challenges. Any idea that "good" families would not be available has simply not been borne out by experience.

Training. The training is designed to impart competence in the core skills needed to provide a therapeutic, home-based milieu for psychiatrically impaired children and adolescents. The development of a clear mission, shared values and cultural heritage, and a common language is crucial to treatment coordination and consistency. The core curriculum includes modules on child development and behavior management and units on analyzing interactions and their probable effects; it fosters positive communication techniques and teaches daily living skills, such as negotiation and conflict resolution. Other topics include therapeutic restraint, modeling, daily record keeping, stress management, human development and sexuality, chemical and substance abuse, physical and mental illness, psychopharmacology, and youth empowerment and advocacy. This model is described in the ABC Training Program by People Places, Inc. (Bryant et al. 1968/1991), and it has been implemented and well received in a number of publicly funded therapeutic foster home programs around the country. It is behaviorally oriented and can be productively supplemented with psychodynamic understanding of, and interventions tailored to, meeting each child's unique background and experiences (Rosenfeld and Wasserman 1990).

Matching.   The clinical team pays careful attention to matching each child's needs with the foster parents' interests, needs, and abilities. One to three preplacement visits should be made so prospective foster children and therapeutic foster parents can test out whether they feel the placement can be viable. Then the child ought to be gradually introduced into the foster family's life (Fine 1993).

Supervision.   A case manager specializing in foster family work oversees, supports, and consults with the therapeutic foster parents and interfaces directly with the child's birth family. The case manager's direct contacts are supplemented by the multidisciplinary team, which is available as needed to support the therapeutically trained foster family for purposes of goal setting, case review, respite, and crisis intervention.

A unique feature that distinguishes therapeutic foster care programs is the team's ability to participate directly, when needed, in the foster family's day-to-day life. This participation can include respite, recreational outings, independent living preparation, birth family visitation, and so on. The program has regular foster parent meetings to discuss each child's ongoing situation, to teach, and to give foster parents an opportunity to share experiences and insights with one another and with staff. This model would review cases at 30-day intervals. The time frame would provide intensive support and consultation to the foster parents and would dramatically tighten and refine goal setting for the patient to enhance treatment and monitor costs more closely. The foster families also have a foster parent peer supervision group that allows parents to network. Fine (1993) found that foster families helped each other with baby-sitting, respite care, and crisis resolution and constructed an extensive list of resources from their combined knowledge about the community.

If the child can return to his or her biological family, this process should begin at the onset of placement. If not, a transfer to publicly funded foster care needs to be arranged. This can become difficult and problematic because, when the foster family has successfully been therapeutic, the foster family members must transfer the child to someone else, breaking ties with a child they have grown to love. It remains to be determined where the therapeutic responsibilities of managed care companies end and the obligations of the public sector begin.

Respite. An alliance with a psychiatric hospital, residential treatment center, or other more highly staffed facility for respite care in emergencies is essential. Because the therapeutic foster home is available, these hospitalizations or respite stays will usually be very brief.

Conclusion

Managed care companies and foster care agencies now share a common interest. We trust that the services we have described and the therapeutic foster home program we have proposed will help foster a dialogue as well as an attempt to find mutually beneficial arrangements.

References

American Psychiatric Association: Diagnostic and Statistical Manual of Mental Disorders, 4th Edition. Washington, DC, American Psychiatric Association, 1994

Bryant B, Snodgrass RD, Houff JK, et al: Parenting Skills Training (1968). Staunton, VA, People Places, 1991

Fine P: A Developmental Network Approach to Therapeutic Foster Care. Washington, DC, Child Welfare League of America, 1993

Rosenfeld AA, Wasserman S: Healing the Heart. Washington, DC, Child Welfare League of America, 1990

Rosenfeld AA, Altman R, Alfaro J, et al: Foster care, child abuse and neglect, and termination of parental rights. Child and Adolescent Psychiatr Clin North Am 3:877–893, 1994

10 Residential Treatment Centers for Youth

William E. Stone, M.D.

Danny is a 14-year-old boy who was referred for residential treatment after spending 10 days in an acute-care psychiatric hospital. This had been his second admission to the hospital in 6 months, each admission being precipitated by a suicide attempt. Subsequent to the first hospitalization, he had been referred to a partial hospital program but refused to attend, and the parents were unable or unwilling to become engaged in the treatment program.

Danny had always had trouble with people in authority, particularly teachers. Frequently during the past 2 years, he had been truant from school, where his grades had been deteriorating; he had been "hanging around" with a group of kids who were known to use drugs; and his parents reported that he was unmanageable at home because of his defiance and irritability. It was reported that he frequently left the house without permission and on one occasion had disappeared for 3 days. His recent hospitalization occurred after a suicide attempt in which he drank a pint of vodka and took a "handful of downers." This episode followed one of many family arguments, but on this occasion the stepfather demanded that Danny be sent to live with his natural father as the stepfather would not put up with him any longer.

According to the history obtained from the family, Danny was the second of two children. His parents moved frequently due to the father's employment as an oil rigger. Both parents were young and unprepared for the demands of raising two boys. Danny had been quite hyperactive when he was younger but had responded well to medication, which was apparently discontinued after a couple of years. Danny was often argumentative with his teachers but had managed to get passing grades. His parents divorced when he was 8 years old, with custody being granted to the mother. Immediately after the divorce, the father remarried and moved away. Danny was very upset, stating that he hated his stepmother and refused to visit their home. When his mother remarried a year later, Danny initially seemed to be very pleased with his new stepfather, but that relationship began to deteriorate after a few months. The stepfather believed in strict discipline and frequently was in conflict with his wife about what he felt was her lack of control over Danny and his 16-year-old brother. Both parents were known to be heavy drinkers, and the stepfather was reported to be occasionally physically abusive when drunk. Danny's mother was under the care of a physician for "chronic depression" and had recently stopped drinking after being placed on medication. The older brother was described as a "real jock" who was out of the house most of the time. He was involved in many sports activities to the obvious satisfaction of his stepfather. Danny and his brother had never been very close.

Danny had been seeing a psychotherapist sporadically before the first suicide attempt and subsequent hospitalization. The therapist reported that the boy had shown evidence of a chronic depression but was difficult to engage in therapy and had not had a very significant response to a trial of antidepressant medication. During the course of the most recent hospital treatment, Danny had been placed on another antidepressant and was no longer considered to be acutely suicidal. He was still very pessimistic about his future but had begun to participate in group psychotherapy with other adolescents. Although he remained somewhat isolated, he appeared to be stable enough to continue his treatment at a lesser level of care. The parents both acknowledged their frustration over managing Danny and indicated a willingness to participate in the treatment, although the stepfather had reservations that it would be of any use.

The evaluation of Danny's case following his admission to the residential treatment center (RTC) indicated that he met the clinical criteria for this level of care and could be expected to profit from 3–5 months of residential treatment. Through diagnostic interviews and psychological testing, it was determined that Danny was suffering from a chronic depressive disorder. It was hypothesized that his antisocial and antagonistic behavior was a reaction to feeling abandoned and betrayed by all of the important adults in his life.

Danny's hyperactivity, which was diagnosed as attention-deficit/hyperactivity disorder, had been present since early childhood. His social adjustment had always been marginal, and he found it impossible to conform to the rigid expectations of his stepfather. His mother, who was quite passive, had never been able to achieve a satisfactory balance between the demands of her second husband and the needs of her troubled son. Her own struggle with depression and alcohol abuse further contributed to the family's dysfunction. Danny's choice of a deviant peer group signaled his despair at ever being able to gain acceptance within his family or the community. As the pressure to conform became more intense, he reacted by increasingly self-destructive activities—even to the point of attempting suicide.

RTCs are designed to provide longer-term treatment to children and adolescents who are sufficiently stable psychiatrically to benefit from a more open environment than that of a hospital.

RTCs have emerged as a level of care in the continuum of mental health services only after many years of confusion about the distinctions between social habilitation and psychiatric treatment. The group home or the residential concept of care has been evolving in the United States since the early 1900s. Historically, both the philosophy and structure of RTCs have varied. Orphanages were developed for abandoned infants, children, and adolescents; rehabilitation centers were developed for mentally retarded persons; and training schools were developed for delinquent youth. As a result of deinstitutionalization, a large number of "group care facilities" have emerged over the past 20 years. Although these institutions were established for the residential care, treatment, and training of children and adolescents, the types of services provided by each have varied widely.

In the early 1970s, the federal government became a major influence in determining what constituted a psychiatric RTC. The Department of Defense, in an effort to manage its Civilian Health and Medical Programs for the Uniformed Services (CHAMPUS) benefit, was particularly concerned about controlling costs and verifying the medical necessity and appropriateness of residential treatment. Eventually, in February 1982, the medical director of CHAMPUS and representatives of mental health professional organizations worked together to develop parameters for the residential treatment of children and adolescents. One of the first efforts of this multidisciplinary group was to develop a working definition of an RTC. In addition to the definition, the group delineated admission criteria and outlined the essential contents of the patient's medical record. The definition of an RTC, and the respective admission and continued stay criteria, differentiated residential care from educational, custodial, and domiciliary care. In recent years, the CHAMPUS definition has become the industry standard for third-party reimbursement for this level of care. Two decades of study and planning have gone into this effort.

CHAMPUS defines an RTC as

A facility, or distinct part of a facility, that provides to children and adolescents under the age of 21, a total, 24-hour therapeutically planned group living and learning situation where distinct and individualized psychotherapeutic interventions can take place. Residential treatment is a specific level of care to be differentiated from acute, intermediate and long-term hospital care, where the least restrictive environment is maintained to allow for normalization of the patient's surroundings. The RTC must be both physically and programmatically distinct if it is a part or subunit of a larger treatment program. An RTC is organized and professionally staffed to provide residential treatment of mental disorders to children and adolescents who have sufficient intellectual potential to respond to active treatment (that is, for whom medical opinion or medical evidence can reasonably conclude that treatment of the mental disorder will result in an improved ability to function outside the RTC), for whom outpatient, partial hospitalization or other level of inpatient treatment is not appropriate and for whom a protected and structured environment is medically or psychologically necessary. (CHAMPUS 1985, p. 8.1.1)

With the advent of managed care, closer scrutiny of medical necessity and lengths of stay at all levels of care has been reflected in significant changes in residential treatment. No longer are patients expected to remain in RTCs for years of treatment, which was typical when social habilitation was the classic model. In the current culture, the length of stay is usually less than 6 months, and patients are transferred to a lesser level of care as soon as it is determined that a 24-hour program is no longer necessary for progress in treatment to continue. Treatment services have been intensified, with a resultant increase in the numbers as well as the qualifications of professional staff.

Patients who are appropriate for the residential level of care must have a psychiatric condition that is both *persistent* and *pervasive.* Their disorder must have been evident over months or years and must be affecting all major areas of their lives (i.e., home, school, community). In the case of Danny, his history indicated that his major symptoms had been evident for a period of at least 3 years. His problems were reflected in his disputes with his family, his involvement with a delinquent peer group, and his poor school performance and attendance. He had not responded well to partial hospital or outpatient therapy, but while hospitalized, he had become sufficiently stable to continue his treatment in a residential setting.

Treatment planning in an RTC is an interdisciplinary as well as multidisciplinary process. No other level of care is able to incorporate such a broad range of therapeutic modalities in an organized plan of treatment. Psychiatrists, psychologists, social workers, nurses, recreation therapists, mental health counselors, and teachers actively participate as members of treatment teams.

Danny's treatment plan at the RTC was directed toward helping him to understand the factors and events in his life that led to his depression while ensuring his safety in this new environment. Goals were also established for the family to improve communications, develop more effective conflict resolution skills, and provide better support for Danny as he worked through his anger and sadness.

Although long-term treatment goals may be identified, it is necessary for the RTC to define those specific criteria that must be met before discharge for continued treatment at another level of care. First, it was important for Danny's family, including the brother, to recognize the extent of the family dysfunction and the role that each person played in perpetuating the pathological interaction. Second, Danny's anger would have to be under better control so that he did not continually defy his stepfather's authority at every point of conflict. Third, the parents would have to agree to establish reasonable rules, expectations, and problem-solving strategies. Finally, it would also be necessary for Danny to tolerate the structure of a public school setting so that his educational development could proceed. The entire family could benefit from the treatment through the support of a consistent therapeutic milieu and an integrated program of medical, psychological, educational, and recreational services.

Residential treatment is categorized as a lesser level of care than inpatient hospitalization because of the open surroundings and the acuity level of the typical patient. It should not, however, be considered to be a less intensive level of treatment. An RTC is professionally staffed 24 hours per day, 7 days per week, and provides a full range of therapy services, including medical care and necessary medication management; individual, group, and family psychotherapy; activity therapy; and educational therapy. In addition to these fundamental treatment elements, most RTCs provide specialized treatment tracks for patients with special needs. These may include programs for patients who are substance abusers, victims of physical or sexual abuse, or perpetrators of abuse.

Although some RTCs are located in a section of a larger facility, such as a hospital, the majority of RTCs in the United States are cottage or campus style. This provides an environment that is less austere and facilitates the normal activities of children and adolescents. Typically, the RTC has living units that may separate the patients by age or sex, classrooms for the educational program, and indoor and outdoor areas for recreation and other activities.

The size and complexity of the program determine the staffing that is required, but, at the very least, the program must have an administrator, a psychiatrist who serves as medical director, professionally qualified psychotherapists, a teacher, an activity therapist, and sufficient nurses and child care workers to provide 24-hour supervision of the milieu.

The overall clinical responsibility for the program is vested in the medical director, who should be a qualified, if not board-certified, child and adolescent psychiatrist. Additional clinical management staff may be employed as program directors or supervisors, depending on the size and complexity of the program. Clinical psychologists and clinical social workers usually provide individual, group, and family therapy; nurses and child care workers primarily are responsible for the management of the milieu. Each patient must be under the care of a psychiatrist who is a member of the professional staff of the organization. Some facilities have an open staff model for medical care, but most RTCs utilize a closed staff model to ensure consistency and active support of the overall program. It is essential that the psychiatrists participate actively in the assessment and treatment planning processes, prescribe any medications that may be needed, provide the oversight of the patient's response to the various therapeutic interventions, and provide support and direction to the staff assigned to the patient's treatment.

At the residential level of care, special treatment procedures such as mechanical restraint and seclusion are considered extraordinary behavioral interventions. Patients at this level of care should be sufficiently stable so that they do not require such extreme measures. Staff are trained in behavioral intervention techniques that encourage verbal rather than physical control. At times of crisis, physical holds may be employed, or the patient may be separated from the group by the use of a quiet room or other area of the facility to regain control of his or her behavior. In recent years, acute-care hospital stays have been shortened, and this has resulted in patients being referred for residential treatment who show more acute symptomatology than was typical in times past. Consequently, RTCs must be prepared to provide a program that meets the needs of impulsive, aggressive, and unpredictable youth. Many patients may require a more gradual transition to this less restrictive environment.

In most cases, patients entering an RTC may have been treated as outpatients, in a partial hospitalization program, or in an acute-care hospital before being referred. Admissions are planned for this level of care, and most states do not license RTCs to accept emergency admissions. The RTC is expected to obtain necessary information about the patient's clinical picture and past psychiatric treatment *before* acceptance to ensure that RTC treatment is appropriate and medically necessary and that the facility has the program and resources to provide for this particular patient. A physician member of the staff must be involved in the decision to approve the patient for admission.

Within 24 hours of admission, the patient should have a medical history and physical examination, a psychiatric evaluation that includes a current mental status, and a nursing assessment. Within the first week, other evaluations are done, including complete psychosocial, psychological, educational, activity, and nutritional assessments. If these required assessments have been completed within a reasonable time before admission, the appropriate clinician can review and endorse the earlier assessment and have it incorporated into the current clinical record. Particular attention should be paid to recording a comprehensive developmental assessment that includes a summary of the patient's developmental history and current level of functioning from the physical, cognitive, social, educational, and psychological perspectives. Because children and adolescents who have a significant emotional disorder can be expected to have some interruption in the process of development, this assessment is of particular importance in determining the most effective treatment approach.

When the assessments are completed, a clinical summary is developed that incorporates and interprets the major findings. This summary designates the principal problems to be treated as well as the focus and strategies to be employed. Treatment plans must be interdisciplinary in this setting. It is particularly important that the treatment team have a consistent approach and that elements such as education and activities therapy be incorporated in the treatment plan. The plan also must include the expectations for both observation and intervention by child care workers, who, by the nature of their assignments, spend the greatest number of hours with the patients in any given day. In a 24-hour-a-day, 7-day-a-week treatment program that may extend over several months, every member of the staff will have contact to a greater or lesser extent with every patient. Consequently, the treatment plan must be comprehensive to ensure a consistency in treatment approach with a careful articulation of those problems that require special attention on the part of the staff.

One of the distinguishing features of the RTC is the emphasis on program. Patients are not admitted to the care of a particular individual clinician as they may be in a hospital environment. The RTC provides a total living situation that is designed to accommodate all of the child's or adolescent's developmental as well as therapeutic needs. Staff members serve as role models and frequently act as parent surrogates during the course of treatment.

Because education is such a critical part of a child's development, RTCs incorporate an active accredited school program within a therapeutic context. Patients attend classes 5 days a week that are conducted by teachers certified in special education. Most RTCs offer a 12-month course of academic instruction to meet educational needs because most patients who are admitted to an RTC have histories of poor or erratic school performance. Vocational services may also be provided. Therapeutic recreation and other activity therapies are scheduled on a daily basis to provide skills training and to enhance group participation and self-esteem. The use of community resources also helps to develop self-help, survival, and basic social skills.

Children who are placed in RTCs require reassurance from the staff that they will not be abused, overlooked, or abandoned. In this setting, individual psychotherapy is provided for all patients. The frequency of therapy varies but should not be less than once a week. Group therapy is also important and is usually provided several times a week. RTCs offer many different types of groups that range from insight-oriented process groups to specialized groups for patients with special issues to address in their treatment. Problem-solving activities are incorporated in every patient's treatment program according to each one's individual needs.

The participation of the family in the treatment program is essential to the patient's success. Family therapy should be a mandatory requirement in every residential treatment program. If the patient's own family either is unwilling or unable to be involved in the treatment, a legally responsible adult must be a participant. The frequency of family therapy should never be less than once per month and more often as needed. For geographically distant families, some facilities provide living accommodations for family treatment weekends. Additional support for families may be provided through the provision of parenting classes, parent support groups, and weekend retreats to help with the development of relationship-building, communication, and problem-solving skills.

The success of an RTC program depends on the integration of all of its elements and the cohesion and competence of its staff. Most of the patients in residential treatment have had serious disruptions in their lives and often have been exposed to very dysfunctional family situations. For these children, a consistent and caring environment that respects their individual differences while providing both treatment and structure can prepare them for a return to a noninstitutional setting. Residential treatment continues to have a significant place in the range of treatment resources. Most patients who are referred for RTC care have had multiple treatment failures in other settings, with a continuing decline in their level of functioning. Experience has demonstrated that this decline often can be interrupted with active interventions that address the combination of developmental and psychopathological factors.

Reference

Civilian Health and Medical Programs for the Uniformed Services: CHAMPUS Policy Manual, Vol 2. CHAMPUS, 1985

Additional Readings

Evangelakis MG: A Manual for Residential and Day Treatment of Children. Springfield, IL, Charles C Thomas, 1974

Lyman RD, Prentice-Dunn S, Gabel S: Residential Treatment of Children and Adolescents. New York, Plenum, 1989

Trieschman A, Whittaker J, Brendtro L: The Other 23 Hours: Child Care Work in a Therapeutic Milieu. Chicago, IL, Aldine 1969

Wells K: Placement of emotionally disturbed children in residential treatment: a review of placement criteria. Am J Orthopsychiatry 61:339–347, 1991

Whittaker J: Caring for Troubled Children: Residential Treatment in a Community Context. San Francisco, CA, Jossey-Bass, 1979

11 Alternative Treatment Services for Children and Adolescents

Alan A. Axelson, M.D.

Mrs. J called the InterCare Patient Access Service. She inquired about services for her 16-year-old son, who had been suspended from school the previous day for fighting with a peer and for possession of marijuana. Mrs. J stated that the problems started this summer and have deteriorated. The school has requested that Sam be evaluated before he returns to class. The call manager took the necessary information and scheduled a family appointment for 3:30 P.M. that day at the Child and Adolescent Assessment Program at InterCare Southwood Psychiatric Hospital.

The author acknowledges the contribution of Thomas Perrone, L.S.W., Director of Alternative Services, InterCare Southwood, in the preparation of this chapter.

Sam stated that he feels a great hopelessness. He is experiencing increased irritability, decreased sleep, early morning awakening, decreased appetite, poor concentration, and social withdrawal. Sam said that he has had a death wish for about 2 months and currently has a plan to kill himself by using a gun. Last night he looked for and found a loaded gun kept by his father. When his brother came into the room, Sam was able to hide the gun before his brother saw it. Sam acknowledges use of marijuana and alcohol. While his parents were with the evaluator, Sam met with a drug and alcohol counselor to assess his chemical usage. The assessment found limited usage of marijuana and alcohol but saw Sam at high risk for continued usage and recommended drug and alcohol educational intervention. Because of the clear plan and means to kill himself, Sam was admitted to the inpatient unit to treat his current depression and to assess further the seriousness of his suicidal behavior.

The inpatient treatment team meeting, held on the third day of hospitalization, was attended by a partial hospitalization liaison staff member. The team recommended that Sam attend the partial hospital program after discharge from the inpatient unit. A children and youth services caseworker and a probation officer were involved and agreed with the recommendation. The managed care company also agreed, providing partial hospitalization would shorten the inpatient treatment phase. Sam was started on antidepressant medication. After 5 days, his depression had diminished, and he wanted to be discharged. Because Sam was ambivalent about continuing on medication and because the family functioning was marginal, the team was hesitant about discharging him, concerned that Sam would not follow up with further treatment. However, after 2 more days of inpatient treatment, during which Sam interacted with the staff of the partial hospitalization program to facilitate his transition there, he was discharged. His parents were comfortable with the discharge plan because of the supportiveness of staff members of the partial hospitalization program.

Sam began the partial hospitalization program, attending each day for 6.5 hours. The treatment goals that were established in the inpatient program were used and expanded. The program helped him with the acceptance of medications and worked with the family to establish effective communication. After 5 days, Sam began integration back to the classroom with a meeting at his school. The school was represented by the counselor and the InterCare in-school social worker. The meeting also included the outpatient therapist, the children and youth services caseworker, the probation officer, Sam, and his parents. The ongoing involvement of the InterCare in-school social worker helped the school staff deal with their concerns about Sam's early return to school.

After successfully integrating attending school, and with his depression under control, Sam continued with outpatient therapy with support from the in-school social worker. The intensity and duration of outpatient therapy was reduced through the support of the in-school social worker. The probation officer helped the family maintain structure.

This vignette describes a consistent and coordinated system of care that serves the family with a continuum of program services and with the cooperation of community agencies. Effective alternative services systems are designed to provide timely, appropriate, integrated, acute behavioral health services for children and adolescents. The key characteristics of these programs are accomplished through teamwork, where each member of the team can count on the availability and responsiveness of other program components and staff. It begins with a central point of contact that is readily available to patient or family member, referring physician, school counselor, or outpatient therapist. A trained patient access specialist can identify and document the level of urgency described by the caller and obtain initial information that can support the work of the professional who provides the initial evaluation. It is important that both the call manager and the assessment staff know the range of resources available to them and be able to respond to issues like geographic convenience, complicated payment contracts, and patient or family resistance.

As indicated in the vignette, a situation that may initially present as a conflict between an adolescent and school can, after assessment, be redefined as involving an array of problems from serious drug and alcohol abuse to very dangerous suicidal behavior. The array of services available to the assessment professional at InterCare Behavioral Health Services and other comprehensive programs includes the following:

- *Ongoing assessment and outpatient treatment.* Assessment and outpatient treatment occur one to two times per week.
- *School liaison and support services.* These services are provided through the Evaluation Prevention Intervention Consultants (EPIC) school-based program.
- *Intensive outpatient program.* This is a structured program of group, individual, and family therapy focused either on drug and alcohol problems or adolescent management problems.
- *Partial hospital programs.* These programs are 5 days per week, 6 hours per day, with either mental health or substance abuse treatment tracks.
- *Twenty-three-hour crisis assessment.* When, in an emergency, the patient's condition is too unstable to be managed in the home setting, the patient is admitted to an inpatient program for up to 23 hours. The goal is to determine the level of stability and the appropriate program for continuing treatment (e.g., inpatient program, partial hospital program, or other alternative level of care).
- *Focused inpatient treatment.* Patients who are dangerous to themselves or someone else or who have a serious psychiatric illness complicated by family instability require intensive 24-hour treatment initiated in the inpatient milieu. The most efficient program is one integrated with an alternative care system that focuses on tasks specifically requiring inpatient interventions. Patients are moved to a partial hospital program or outpatient program as soon as feasible.

To achieve the level of integration necessary to make a truly effective system, treatment must be internally managed and coordinated by a treatment team that is confident and empowered to work with the patient and the family. The patient and family ca.1 enter into a stable treatment relationship within an integrated treatment process. Uncertainty about the points of transition or the availability of the next treatment resource brings instability to the treatment process. This often leads to a breakdown in the transition from inpatient to partial hospital treatment, with treatment failing to progress past the crisis intervention stage. The latter can lead to continued developmental dysfunction for the child or adolescent and at times recidivism, resulting in the patient's reentering higher-intensity treatment at some later time.

Continuum of Care

The concept of a continuum of care is not a recent development. It was discussed the first time at the White House Conference on Children in 1909. The concept was later recommended by the Joint Commission on Mental Health of Children in 1969 and, more recently, the Child and Adolescent Service System Program. This program focuses on practical planning, improved advocacy, and increased cooperation with parents. In the past two decades, experts (Hobbs 1982; Knitzer 1982; Stroul and Friedman 1986) have highlighted the vast discrepancy between the numbers of children and youth in need of mental health services and those who actually receive services. More than half of these children receive no treatment at all, and many who are treated are receiving inappropriate care (Saxe et al. 1988). The availability of alternative treatment settings plays a role in placing children and adolescents in the most appropriate treatment facility. Knitzer (1982), Behar (1985), and Silver (1984) all reported that approximately 40% of inpatient placements were inappropriate because the children could have been treated in less restrictive settings, if such less restrictive treatment settings were available. This remains the situation despite evidence that even severely emotionally disturbed children can benefit from treatment while living in their own homes when a comprehensive system of care is present in the community (Behar 1985).

Even where services are available, the lack of coordination between programs compromises the effectiveness of the interventions (Saxe et al. 1987; Stroul and Friedman 1986). Given the developmental complexity and multiple needs of children and adolescents, services must be both available and coordinated (Behar 1985) if they are going to be effective.

The concept of a continuum of care stems from the belief that to meet the patients' and families' needs, a treatment system should provide comprehensive services that offer a full array of programs. These often involve services from both the public and private sectors. A continuum must offer an organized and systematic method of planning and delivering those multiple services. This approach attempts to deliver needed services on an individualized basis and in a coordinated manner, relying on case management that assumes responsibility for the integrated treatment programs and facilitates transition between services. It is also designed to be community based, involving various agencies pertinent to the treatment of the patient and family (Stroul and Friedman 1986).

Sufficient family, educational, and social supports, working in cooperation with mental health and medical treatment facilities, are vital for the treatment of our children. The appropriate diagnosis and effective treatment of psychiatric illnesses can have a profound effect on the child or adolescent making a transition into an adult, self-sustaining role because young people are in the midst of dealing with so many developmental issues. The ability of psychiatric treatment to provide a vehicle for the restoration of the developmental trajectory can be achieved only if the necessary resources are accessible and applied in a timely fashion.

The availability of a comprehensive system of care will have multiple effects on the child and on the child's world. The skillful treatment of an adjustment disorder or a single episode of depression not only relieves the suffering of the individual, but also often positively affects the way the family views the patient and alters the way they interact. This positive effect is even more apparent with recurring and persistent problems. The suffering of the patients, their capacity to be cooperative partners in treatment, their utilization of resources, and their productivity will be affected for years to come. In developing treatment services for children and adolescents, it is important that we clearly understand that a treatment continuum for adults and a continuum for children and adolescents need to different because the goals are different. The relief of symptoms and restoration of the previous level of functioning, often the treatment objectives in a managed care environment, are insufficient for children and adolescents. Because children are engaged in a process of rapid, continuous change, ill-timed or insufficient treatment can permanently disrupt a child's relationship with the educational process or capacity for positive social relationships. Adults who have achieved a level of stability before a psychiatric illness are more likely to respond to limited interventions. With each child, there must be a focus on restoring developmental trajectory. The ability to achieve this restoration depends on a service continuum that allows the child to be treated with the appropriate level of service, with sufficient length and intensity of intervention. Follow-up must actively address the child's developmental functions.

Levels of Care

Because of the variety of alternative programs that have been developed, and because each program has unique services and staffing, it is very difficult to categorize and define them. The American Association for Partial Hospitalization has been working on this issue and recommends three levels describing the continuum of ambulatory mental health services between inpatient and outpatient care (see Tables 11–1, 11–2, and 11–3). The association focuses on variables related to the programs, including the function and intensity of the program, as well as important characteristics such as medical involvement, location of the treatment milieu, level of structure, and locus of responsibility and control.

These descriptions of levels of care by an organization that enjoys strong support in the treatment community are an important step toward standardizing the terms necessary to evaluate clinical decisions and outcomes. Although these descriptions have good face validity, translating them into actual clinical programs and matching the criteria of the various managed care organizations to these levels of treatment are processes that will take considerable time.

In developing levels of care necessary to treat psychiatric and substance abuse problems fully, it is important to differentiate between patients who require acute treatment and those for whom it is clear that brief, time-limited therapies are going to have only a short-term impact. Up to the present time, this differentiation has often been made economically by making the private insured system responsive to the acute treatment needs. Once it has been determined that the patient's problems are severe and persistent, the patient's care becomes the responsibility of a publicly funded program or some other special category. The movement of managed care into the Medicaid arena challenges us to establish program descriptions and placement criteria for services beyond the relatively brief treatments considered under the managed care medical necessity criteria for psychiatric treatment. Substance abuse, as well as some medical and surgical illnesses, have well-established criteria for differentiating acute medical care from rehabilitation. Psychiatric treatment should also develop this rehabilitation perspective, identifying certain residential and community-based programs as having rehabilitation objectives. Admission criteria and continuing stay criteria should be determined from that perspective. A rehabilitative focus is indicated when psychiatric dysfunction persists and interferes with education and socialization. It is also

Table 11–1. Patient and service variables across the continuum

Service variable	Definition
Program function	Refers to the specific patient care mission of the services
Scheduled programming	Planned hours of treatment
Structure	Routines, scheduled activities, expectations, and special treatment procedures integral to nonhospital-based services
Milieu	Cohesive, consistent, therapeutic environment, created either within a program or community or through coordination of people, space, materials, equipment, and activities
Crisis availability	Crisis intervention and emergency services describing the blanket of protective services that cover the patient during nontreatment hours
Medical involvement	Degree of responsibility and participation assumed by medical and nursing personnel
Accessibility	Mechanisms by which a new patient makes contact and is able to begin treatment; intake and admission procedures
Responsibility and control	Role of treating professionals in providing a safety net for the patient

Patient variable	Definition
Level of functioning	Patient's ability to perform the various tasks of daily living
Psychiatric signs and symptoms	Patient's presenting problems and requisite assessment of suicidal/homicidal tendencies, thought processes, and orientation
Risk/dangerousness	Degree of jeopardy present secondary to the patient's psychiatric illnesses, including dangerousness to self and others, need for confinement, and potential for escalation of symptoms
Commitment to treatment/follow through	Patient's ability to comprehend and accomplish the tasks necessary to benefit from treatment at a specified level of care

(continued)

Table 11–1. Patient and service variables across the continuum
(continued)

Patient variable	Definition
Social support system	Patient's ability to ask for, use, and accept assistance provided by family members or community supports

Source. Reprinted from American Association for Partial Hospitalization, Inc., *The Continuum of Ambulatory Behavioral Healthcare Services,* 1995. Used with permission.

necessary when families have difficulty maintaining a developmentally supportive environment with additional resources.

Staffing Issues

Organizations will need to look at staffing profiles in the continuum of care. Short- and long-term residential programs, partial hospitalization programs, and intensive outpatient programs are all heading toward staffing with master's-prepared social workers and bachelor's-level staff providing the majority of direct services. Culhane et al. (1994) discussed staffing issues in a partial hospitalization program. They described master's-level counselors and social workers and bachelor's-level mental health workers as constituting the core full-time service staffs. Culhane et al. used percentages to discuss staffing patterns. Table 11–4 reflects their numbers changed to ratios per 15-patient census. This is evident in our own partial programs.

The effective use of part-time psychiatrists and psychologists relies on the clear communication between the staff and the professionals who are not there on a full-time basis. The shared information must be accurate, and the staff must have sound clinical judgment. There must be an atmosphere of continuing consultation and training to be sure that the whole team works together.

Table 11–2. The continuum of ambulatory behavioral health care services: service variables

	Ambulatory level 1	Ambulatory level 2	Ambulatory level 3
Service function	Crisis stabilization and acute symptom reduction; serves as alternative to and prevention of hospitalization	Stabilization, symptom reduction, and prevention of relapse	Coordinated treatment for prevention of decline in functioning where outpatient services cannot adequately meet patient need
Scheduled programming	Minimum of 4 hours/ day scheduled and intensive treatment over 4–7 days	Minimum of 3–4 hours/ day, at least 2–3 days/week	A minimum of 4 hours/ week
Crisis backup availability	An organized and integrated system of 24-hour crisis backup with immediate access to current clinical and treatment information	A 24-hour crisis and consultation service	A 24-hour crisis and consultation service
Medical involvement	Medical supervision	Medical consultation	Medical consultation available
Accessibility	Capable of admitting within 24 hours	Capable of admitting within 48 hours	Capable of admitting within 72 hours

(continued)

Table 11–2. The continuum of ambulatory behavioral health care services: service variables (*continued*)

	Ambulatory level 1	Ambulatory level 2	Ambulatory level 3
Milieu	Preplanned, consistent, and therapeutic; primarily within treatment setting	Active therapeutic within both treatment setting and home and community	Active therapeutic; primarily within home and community
Structure	High degree of structure and scheduling	Regularly scheduled, individualized	Individualized and coordinated
Responsibility and control	Staff aggressively monitors and supports patient and family	Monitoring and support shared with patient, family, and support system	Monitoring and support placed primarily with patient, family, and support system
Service examples	Partial hospitalization programs	Psychosocial rehabilitation	Multimodal outpatient services
	Day treatment programs	Intensive outpatient programs	Aftercare
	Intensive in-home crisis intervention	Behavioral aides	Clubhouse programs
	Outpatient detoxification services	Assertive community treatment	In-home services
	23-hour observation beds	23-hour respite beds	

Source. Reprinted from American Association for Partial Hospitalization, Inc., *The Continuum of Ambulatory Behavioral Healthcare Services*, 1995. Used with permission.

Table 11–3. The continuum of ambulatory behavioral health care services: patient variables

	Ambulatory level 1	Ambulatory level 2	Ambulatory level 3
Level of functioning	Severe impairment in multiple areas of daily life	Marked impairment in at least one area of daily life	Moderate impairment in at least one area of daily life
Psychiatric signs and symptoms	Severe to disabling symptoms related to acute condition or exacerbation of severe/persistent disorder	Moderate to severe symptoms related to acute condition or exacerbation of severe/persistent disorder	Moderate symptoms related to acute condition or exacerbation of severe/persistent disorder
Risk/danger-ousness	Marked instability and/or dangerousness with high risk of confinement	Moderate instability and/or dangerousness with some risk of confinement	Mild instability with limited dangerousness and low risk of confinement
Commitment to treatment/follow through	Inability to form more than initial treatment contract requires close monitoring and support	Limited ability to form extended treatment contract requires frequent monitoring and support	Ability to sustain treatment contract with intermittent monitoring and support
Social support system	Impaired ability to access or use caretaker, family, or community support	Limited ability to form relationships or seek support	Ability to form and maintain relationships outside of treatment

Source. Reprinted from American Association for Partial Hospitalization, Inc., *The Continuum of Ambulatory Behavioral Healthcare Services,* 1995. Used with permission.

Table 11–4. Staff time per 15-patient census, by staff position

Positions	Staff time per 15-patient census	Positions	Staff time per 15-patient census
Psychiatrists	0.39	Registered nurses	0.38
Other physicians	0.03	Other registered nurses	0.84
Psychologists	0.31	Teachers	0.67
Master's-level counselors	1.21	Other mental health workers (B.A.)	1.74
Social workers (M.S.W.)	1.00	Other mental health workers (< B.A.)	0.83
Other social workers	0.36	Other physical health workers	0.21
Administrative	1.55		

Source. Reprinted from Culhane DP, Hadley TR, Kiser LJ: "A National Profile of Partial Hospitalization Programs." *Continuum* 1:91, 1994. Used with permission.

Alternative Treatment Locations

Organizing special child and adolescent services in centralized locations, and expecting families to utilize those services, is not sufficient. A methodology that is gaining prominence is in-home service. A team, often a master's-level social worker and a bachelor's-level child mental health specialist, use direct counseling, family support, and therapeutic activities and interactions with the child and family to help reestablish family functioning. They also enhance support systems for children who are experiencing severe problems or living in dysfunctional home situations. Often the in-home services programs are a central part of a "wraparound" service where innovative treatment and support programs, individualized to the needs of the particular child, are able to maintain a very difficult child in his or her home and school.

Parents must support the in-home programs. Sometimes, with resistant parents, entering the home cannot be accomplished. Also, home services are usually reserved for children for whom high-intensity programs are required.

Another effective alternative is day treatment programs associated with approved private schools. A consistent, therapeutic education milieu, comprehensive individual group and family treatment, school attendance requirements, and transportation provide opportunities for growth and rehabilitation to children who otherwise might be in long-term psychiatric hospitals or residential treatment programs.

Another approach effectively used by InterCare for the past 6 years is contracting social workers who are InterCare employees to school districts to work directly within the school setting, providing support and early intervention services. The staff of the EPIC program use their influence with school counselors, teachers, and administrators to enhance the supportive nature of the school environment. In addition, they are very effective as "on the spot" case managers helping a child recently discharged from an inpatient or partial hospital program make the transition back to the classroom. They encourage the child to work in their outpatient program, providing emotional support that supplements the individual and family treatment.

A step beyond the supportive services provided by the EPIC social worker is treatment provided in the school setting. Here, with the formal enrollment in a treatment process, and with permission of the family and child, the benefits of therapeutic activities, group therapy, and individual counseling are available for children who may be too resistant to commit to a partial hospital or outpatient treatment program. Bringing the services into the school and having an impact on how the child and the school interact may address some of the very difficult problems of young people who currently have little opportunity for positive impact in their lives.

Organizational Integration

A cohesive team approach is a vital element of treatments that include higher-intensity services. It is important that this team approach be evident throughout the entire system of care. It will be the organization's responsibility to integrate the treatment in a continuous process where patients move from one treatment level to the next with a sense of continuity and continued focus on treatment goals. This mind-set of a continuous treatment process where there is mutual confidence and reliance is a key factor in good clinical care and cost-effective treatment. Each provider must make the next treatment provider's job as easy as possible, supporting the patient's confidence in each aspect of the continuum of service.

We are all very familiar with the program boundaries and turf issues that can be detrimental to service integration. Although one can attribute this to pettiness or lack of maturity, part of it is very typical of organizational behavior. In taking on the task of developing the continuum of care, the organization must be committed to becoming an integrated system—to approach each day with the challenge of making system integration work. It must nondefensively engage in problem solving when the inevitable breakdowns in communication and continuity occur. When a patient experiences a problem or engages in criticism, there can be a tendency to deflect either clinical or administrative responsibility (e.g., "That's a problem with the billing department; I don't have anything to do with that part of our organization."). To be effective, the system of continuity of care must function as one of mutual responsibility.

Each organization must be prepared to evaluate past performance and systems and procedures, deciding what changes are necessary to enhance patient services. This may entail reviewing current job descriptions and organizational and departmental structures to determine if they still serve the purpose for which they were intended. It is also identifying and abandoning outdated rules and fundamental assumptions that are not consistent with current mental health services. One must be prepared to modify, reduce, or lose some favored treatment components for new, innovative, and more patient-based treatment approaches necessary for growth.

Accessibility

A continuum of care system must have ease of accessibility and must be user-friendly. A comprehensive array of services can be developed that can encompass the entire spectrum of care, but the process of entering that system can be so time consuming and difficult that families and professionals become unwilling to use it. Delaying necessary treatment for a child increases the chance for developmental disruption and complicates the treatment process.

The intake process is a vital element to the success of treatment and to the success of a continuum of care. Hindering access to the system is a limited knowledge on the part of patients and referring professionals regarding the range of available services and the method of access. Parents, physicians, social services agencies, emergency room personnel, and school personnel need to be well informed regarding a simple process for obtaining access to the system. Research indicates that even when there are no financial barriers to entering psychiatric treatment, parents, pediatricians, and other primary care physicians fail to identify and refer children with significant psychiatric problems.

A continuum of care should have one point of access that anyone can use to obtain services. Anyone should be able to call one number, and through that one simple call the process of serving the patient is initiated. The effectiveness and efficiency of treatment systems are enhanced not by keeping people out, but by understanding and shaping their expectations at the point of entry. By connecting them with the treatment resources best designed to respond to their needs, and by helping them understand what they are expected to contribute to the treatment effort, the possibility of positive outcome is greatly increased. Dissatisfaction frequently comes because of unmet expectations, not unmet needs. A cumbersome intake process, designed from the viewpoint of the provider rather than the patient, increases frustration and lowers motivation. Access procedures must be designed from the perspective of patients and others looking in to the program, not the program looking out. In this age of managed care, we must accept that there is a necessary preauthorization process when services with the cost of partial hospitalization or in-home services are utilized. This preauthorization process must be timely. The effective use of the continuum of services depends on each aspect of care following one after another at critical transition points.

Generally, payment is through capitated arrangements or other types of risk-sharing contracts. The next best arrangement is management by a specialized behavioral health utilization company. A sophisticated company can understand the subtleties of treatment, authorizing and monitoring the entire treatment process rather than approving a limited number of days at a particular level of care. Systems that depend on authorization from a primary care physician or special permission from an employer to flex benefits are generally so cumbersome or insensitive that the effectiveness of treatment is reduced. Ineffective treatment often relates to a failure of commitment, on the part of the families and patients, to an ongoing process of outpatient treatment and family systems change.

Funding Availability

As we speak of the need for a continuous care system to treat our young people, we must consider how these services are funded. One of the many obstacles is the lack of support by insurance providers and state and federal funding streams. I have discussed the need for a system to be user-friendly, and this applies to funding sources as well. The need to precertify or have benefits flexed can be a cumbersome process that can delay an admission for hours and, at times, for days. The governmental funding sources have recently initiated alternative ways to access money; however, the process is so difficult and complex that many agencies have refused to attempt to use the funds. This travesty results in patients' and families' losing necessary services and, furthermore, places the health of our children in jeopardy.

As systems of care move toward an integration of services and cooperative efforts with agencies, funding sources must become more flexible and increase their efforts to provide a package of benefits allowing patients to access the necessary system and allowing professionals to use their judgment to determine the appropriate level of care. Payers should consider allocating resources through different methods, finding new ways to utilize the resources that are available and eliminating wasteful spending on unnecessary services.

A new and innovative treatment spectrum cannot survive in a vacuum. It must have the support and resources to facilitate its development. We need insurance coverage that allows professionals to do what they know best and to construct a treatment plan that will maximize the chances of the patient to become well. Regulatory agencies must update and modify the regulations to reflect the treatment programs that are currently being used and not those that are outdated and unrelated.

Special Issues

Alternative services in the continuum of care are wonderful concepts, but problems occur with the practical business of implementing the services. Pilot and demonstration projects, developed with special supports and funding parameters, can look very promising. When these projects are actually implemented, there are structural and program issues that can defeat the most dedicated clinical system. These issues to be considered are in the following categories:

- Patient volume
- Patient and family commitment
- Resource availability
- Coordination and integration

Most alternative programs are group focused. There needs to be a critical mass of patients to make group programs effective and to absorb the fixed costs and administrative overhead associated with all clinical programs. Acute-care programs are characterized by brief lengths of stay. This requires a large volume of admissions to maintain groups of approximately 15 patients, which are necessary to make partial hospital programs and intensive outpatient programs work. From my experience, this requires responsibility for about 200,000 covered lives. There are logistical problems in locating services so that they are geographically convenient to that type of population density. When partial hospital services are underutilized, there can be a tendency on the part of the administration to extend lengths of stay. This extension exactly counters the alignment of incentives that care management programs desire. When programs are fully utilized, costs are held at a reasonable rate and utilizations are appropriate. The same problem with patient volume relates to seasonal variations. Families seek acute psychiatric services for children and adolescents during the school periods, causing serious difficulties in maintaining program viability and staffing on a 12-month basis.

Although there are certainly some families who extend themselves to avoid hospitalization and who welcome alternative services, for many of today's families, strapped by overscheduling and limited resources, inpatient or residential treatment is preferred. Not only are there transportation issues, but to struggle each day with a resistant adolescent, getting him or her to attend a partial hospital program or to be regularly involved in a biweekly intensive outpatient program, requires more energy than some families can muster. From the managed care company's short-range point of view, these issues result in self-exclusion from utilization of the benefit. From a longer-range perspective of supporting the effective development of children and adolescents, a brief episode of crisis intervention, without dealing with the resistance and avoidance that defend against more significant treatment interventions, can result in chronically dysfunctional young adults. For these alternative services to be effective, we must address the issue of engagement of the reluctant adolescent and the exhausted or uninvolved family.

In the new systems of behavioral health care, various types of intensive outpatient services and community-based services will bear the major responsibility for definitive patient treatment. I seriously question if we have evaluated the cost involved in providing the level of services needed. There are certain efficiencies and controls that are available when patients are consistently in one place, such as a residential inpatient program. To approach the intensity of treatment necessary to truly intervene with children and adolescents, higher staffing ratios and high-impact outreach services may be needed.

As we now enter a phase of designing programs and matching them to the needs of patients, we must honestly address and account for all the resources needed to get the job done. Current efforts to develop and support partial hospital programs have used inpatient programs, grants, and institutional resources to subsidize funding. Recently published Civilian Health and Medical Programs for the Uniformed Services (CHAMPUS) rates indicate a fairly common trend of paying at about 50% of inpatient rates (see Table 11–5). This may be appropriate for the level 2–type programs described earlier, where the patients stay for a number of weeks. The resources needed to provide an ambulatory level 1 program, dealing with high-risk patients trying to avoid hospital treatment, can approach three-quarters of the cost of the current regular inpatient rates. As a greater volume of patients move from the traditional inpatient psychiatric hospital setting to the alternative services program, we have to look at the appropriate allocation of resources to meet patient needs

Table 11-5. CHAMPUS rates

Regional specific rates for psychiatric hospitals and units with low CHAMPUS volume		Partial hospitalization rates for full-day and half-day programs		
United States census region	Rate[a]	United States census region	Full day 6+ hrs	Half day 3-5 hrs
Northeast		Northeast		
New England (ME,NH,VT,RI,CT)	$515	New England	$211	$159
Mid Atlantic (NY,NJ,PA)	492	Mid Atlantic	230	173
Midwest		Midwest		
East North Central (OH,IN,IL,MI,WI)	426	East North Central	205	154
West North Central (MN,IA,MO,ND, SD,NE,KS)	402	West North Central	202	152
South		South		
South Atlantic (DE,MD,DC,VA, WV,NC,SC, GA,FL)	509	South Atlantic	218	164
East South Central (KY,TN,AL,MS)	550	East South Central	237	178
West South Central (AR,LA,TX,OK)	463	West South Central	234	176
West		West		
Mountain (MT,ID,WY,CO, NM,AZ,UT,NV)	462	Mountain	243	183
Pacific (WA,OR,CA, AK,HI)	545	Pacific	239	180

[a]The wage portion of the rate, subject to the area wage adjustment, is 71.40%.

Source. Reprinted from The National Association of Psychiatric Health Systems, *CEO Forecast,* No 39, October 14, 1994. Used with permission.

carefully; otherwise, there certainly will be a deterioration of quality in patient care. In a rush toward the deinstitutionalization of state hospital patients, we underestimated the cost of community-based services. It is important that we do not repeat that mistake today as we de-emphasize acute hospital treatment.

To utilize a program of alternative services appropriately depends on an accurate initial assessment, creative treatment planning, and continuity of responsibility. The patient's condition and treatment program must be reevaluated continually. Members of the treatment team must be aware of the clinical resources available and methods of connection.

The key to this whole alternative services approach is coordination. This can be done through very positive consistent working relationships in a network of services. Each component must perform the services that it is specifically assigned to do and prepare the patient for the next part of the treatment program. This coordination is complex and can represent a hidden cost, particularly if the volume of patients drops at the transition points or if patients and families have a sense that they are starting all over as they move from their partial hospital program to their outpatient therapy. Developing integrated systems where a single organizational unit is responsible for a significant part of the alternative services system, coordinating other aspects such as the inpatient treatment and the general outpatient treatment, is one method to achieve the flexibility necessary to deal with issues of patient volume, accessibility, and cost. Integrated medical records and information systems can assist this coordination.

Consistently applying the principles of total quality management throughout the alternative care system is essential to achieve and maintain effective program coordination. Unless the inevitable problems of system fit and interaction are addressed and solved, the patient and family must expend their energies to pull the treatment components together.

As we are developing new systems, we must be very realistic about the part that cost control plays in the overall planning and management process. For the short term, cost can be reduced through a decrease in staffing levels, lower pay for professionals, and withholding services. All of these things have negative effects. Positive direction is toward outcomes-oriented program evaluation, increased productivity, and modification and elimination of tasks that do not contribute to the objectives of the program and patient care. The ideal concept is an integrated system of care that meets the needs of the patient and allows services offered to be accessible and well funded. The system we all are striving to achieve is an individualized treatment service that is not just case managed, but one that is both responsive and responsible. In such a system, the flow of treatment can exist and be used therapeutically. Although it is not specifically crisis oriented, an integrated system of care is adept at dealing with a crisis while focusing on the larger goal of continuous rehabilitation.

A continuum of care in a managed care environment will be successful only if a mind-set of teamwork, integration, alignment, and empowerment occurs. The elements of quality management must work together as a group to deliver services that improve the health of the population. Added to this is the continuing struggle with the ethical dilemmas presented when we are paid to improve the behavioral health care of a community rather than to deliver a day of inpatient treatment or an hour of psychotherapy. These challenges either can restrict access to necessary care or can encourage flexible and innovative treatment approaches.

We must always remain focused on the ultimate goal in developing a continuum of care. That goal is not to save money but to provide a system of care that can contribute to developing healthy children and adolescents for tomorrow.

References

Behar L: Changing patterns of state responsibility: a case study of North Carolina. Journal of Clinical Child Psychology 14:188–199, 1985

Culhane D, Hadley T, Kiser LJ: A national profile of partial hospitalization programs. Continuum 1(2):81–93, 1994
Hobbs N: The Troubled and Troubling Child. San Francisco, CA, Jossey-Bass, 1982
Knitzer J: Unclaimed Children. Washington, DC, Children's Defense Fund, 1982
Saxe L, Cross T, Silverman N, et al: Children's Mental Health: Problems and Treatment. Durham, NC, Duke University Press, 1987
Saxe L, Cross T, Silverman N: Children's mental health: the gap between what we know and what we do. Am Psychol 43:800–807, 1988
Silver AA: Children in classes for the severely emotionally handicapped. J Dev Behav Pediatr 3:49–54, 1984
Stroul B, Friedman R: A System of Care for Severely Emotionally Disturbed Youth. Washington, DC, Child and Adolescent Service System Program Technical Assistance Center, 1986

Additional Readings

Behar L, Macbeth G, Holland J: Distribution and costs of mental health services within a system of care for children and adolescents. Administration and Policy in Mental Health 20:283–294, 1993
Dore M, Wilkinson A, Sonis W: Exploring the relationships between continuum of care and intrusiveness of children's mental health services. Hospital and Community Psychiatry 43:44–48, 1992
England M, Cole R: Building systems of care for youth with serious mental illness. Hospital and Community Psychiatry 43:630–633, 1992
Feldman JL, Fitzpatrick RJ: Managed Health Care. Washington, DC, American Psychiatric Press, 1992
Knitzer J: Children's mental health policy: challenging the future. Journal of Emotional and Behavioral Disorders 1:8–16, 1993
Behar L: Financing mental health services for children and adolescents. Bull Menninger Clin 55:127–139, 1990
Pothier PC: Child mental health problems and policy. Arch Psychiatr Nurs 11:159–169, 1988
Schreter RK, Sharfstein SS, Schreter CA (eds): Allies and Adversaries: The Impact of Managed Care on Mental Health. Washington, DC, American Psychiatric Press, 1994

Tarico V, Low B, Trupin E, et al: Children's mental health services: a parent's perspective. Community Ment Health J 25:313–326, 1989

Tuma J: Mental health services for children: the state of the art. Am Psychol 44:188–199, 1989

12 School-Based Mental Health Programs

Paul Jay Fink, M.D.

I have been involved in the development of mental health programs at three different schools in Philadelphia, one of which is Pierce Middle School. There are approximately 600 students at Pierce; all are African American and live in very difficult and dangerous neighborhoods.

Through the implementation of several different programs at Pierce (which I describe in this chapter), we were able to identify 10 students who needed additional help. I volunteered to pay for their transportation to and from the Belmont Center, also in Philadelphia, for evaluation and treatment, which would be provided pro bono by our staff of residents. Before we could bring the students to Belmont, we needed permission from their parents or legal guardians, and letters were sent. Not one parent responded, which was not too surprising because it is apparent that any child who is in such desperate straits at school has problems that originated at home. Undaunted, I decided to send our residents to Pierce to create a school-based mental health clinic.

177

The residents were welcomed with open arms by the faculty and students and did an excellent job. They worked with students on an individual basis, formed groups, and served as consultants to the school's counselors and teachers.

This experience was uplifting but also depressing, considering the need is so great and a pro bono effort like this does not even begin to scratch the surface of the problem. It does demonstrate, however, that when a school is prepared to address the multitude of problems it faces and has an administration and faculty who are willing to work with mental health professionals, school-based programs can indeed provide vital services for our children and help them to grow and learn.

Schools as Mental Health Providers

For years, social services and health and mental health agencies have tried to bring their services into schools. The purpose is simple: to improve access to care and relieve some of the stress on teachers and students that is brought on by personal, family, and community factors that interfere with and undermine children's ability to learn. I have seen these efforts increase over the last 10 years and watched them become a rallying point for those of us who would like to see a change from our current nonsystem of volunteers and do-gooders to an established system of school-based mental health services.

The concept of full-service schools is that schools should become community centers that stay open well beyond traditional school hours—perhaps even around the clock—to fulfill a variety of needs. In declining communities, the school building has emerged as the one piece of real estate that is publicly owned, centrally located, and used consistently.

Currently, school-based clinics are usually health clinics dealing with epidemiology, immunizations, and identification of (and only recently the treatment of) physical illnesses. Also common in these clinics is an effort to address social issues. In urban poverty pockets, these social issues undermine students' ability to concentrate and maintain interest in what seem like trivial matters (e.g., English, math, history) when compared with the problems and fears they face in real life. The six major epidemics occurring in our schools are pregnancy, HIV, sexually transmitted diseases, violence, child abuse, and drug and alcohol problems. The worse the neighborhood, the more prevalent are these six epidemics. However, even children in the best communities face some of these problems.

Over the years, we have seen an increase in school counselors and psychologists, but, for the most part, they are being used more as guidance counselors than therapists. For example, student assistance programs have been developed primarily to deal with drug and alcohol problems but are generally limited to evaluation. Once an evaluation is completed, getting that child proper care still depends on the willingness of parents to take that child to a mental health or substance abuse treatment center.

Two things are clear. First, schools are where the children (and the problems) are located. Second, mental health professionals must go into the schools not only to evaluate students, but also to treat them and their families for mental illnesses and those problems that will impair the students' mental functions and capacity to learn, grow, and enter the mainstream. Creating mental health service programs in our schools provides continuity of care and more opportunities to learn about a child from a variety of sources, which in turn permits the ability to care for the total child.

History of School-Based Programs

For the past 100 years, the availability of services, particularly health services, has depended on the support of politicians. According to Dryfoos (1994):

> Over the years, the supply of services within schools has been turned on and off. The demand has fluctuated, reflect-

ing the social environment for families. In periods of poverty, unrest, and disadvantage, service provision in the
schools has risen. In periods of relative affluence and in the
absence of new immigration populations, provision has
been limited. The private sector, which authorizes the sup-
ply through policy control, has been willing to allow public
agencies to go into schools during crisis periods (epidemics, economic depressions) but has withdrawn approval
whenever school services loomed as competition. This is
most evident among physicians whose sporadic presence in
school has mirrored the fluctuating approval of the American Medical Association. (p. 41)

The advent of school-based clinics, in lieu of school nurses
and psychologists and other employees of the schools, has only
been in place for a decade. There are currently at least 500 clinics
providing primary mental health care in or near school buildings
for an estimated 500,000 students annually. For the most part,
these clinics are "add-ons." That is, an outside agency comes into
a school and creates a new unit—a clinic or a center that coexists
with the already-in-place educational system. The educational
system will shift as a result of the presence of health and social
services in the school. The shortage of resources, however, always makes for a competitive situation between the educational
needs and the needs of the support services.

According to Dryfoos (1994), "In centers with mental health
personnel, substantial numbers of students and their families
are gaining access to psychosocial counseling that was not available to them within the community. The demand is overwhelming" (p. 135).

At the Balboa High School Teen Health Center in San Francisco, California, it was found that 70% of the diagnoses showed
the need for further intervention for problems such as depression, anxiety, and family problems. It was also found that the
"presence of a nonthreatening confidential adviser apparently
opens up communication about such issues as physical and sexual abuse, parental drug use, and fears of violence" (Dryfoos
1994, pp. 93–94).

James Comer is the best-known proponent of school-based mental health programs that are developed with an understanding of the psychological needs of the children. Comer's (1980) book, *School Power,* describes an intervention project he started in 1968. Over the years, Comer has become a powerful and passionate voice in trying to help people understand that meeting the needs and supporting the values of schools and students are a team effort. According to Comer:

> Our conclusion is that most programs designed to improve schooling fail because they do not adequately address the developmental needs of children and the potential for conflict in the relationship between home and school, among school staff, and among school staff and students. They do not consider the structural arrangements, specific skills, and conditions school people need to address the complexities of today's schools. (p. 38)

To involve administrators, teachers, students, and families, Comer (1980) developed the concept of "process," which has been copied throughout the country. His team from the Yale University Child Study Center went into two schools with a demonstration project and showed how difficult it was to get all of the political elements in the school to participate openly and actively in the best interests of the children. To turn this around, Comer included all the involved parties. He used parents as decision makers and got them to come into the school other than when their children were in trouble. Parents became "helpers" in the classroom. According to Comer, the strength of his program comes from focusing on the needs of the entire school rather than one particular area of concern. Institutional change rather than individual change is what Comer recommends.

In many ways, Comer's (1980) ideas paved the way for our current efforts (in Philadelphia) to develop full-service community schools. The idea to provide a multitude of services so that various elements of the community can come together in a single place—the school—with the best interest of the community at heart and the understanding that children are an essential part of the community's future, is not very different from Comer's philosophy. However, the community school concept, which I endorse, tackles the problem differently from Comer's concept of process in that it eliminates (at least for now) the very important but difficult, tedious, and politically nerve-racking efforts to get the entire community to join, understand, and participate in a helpful way.

Without an overall organized program in place, what we see today are hundreds of individuals entering schools. For example, the principal may invite someone in to initiate a program, the guidance counselor invites someone else in to work on a different program, and a teacher invites a third person in to address a problem he or she might face. The result is several programs that address issues such as AIDS, substance abuse, or pregnancy, without any integration.

This is not to diminish in any way the commitment or accomplishments of these do-gooders. In fact, in some measure, this is how I became involved with the school district of Philadelphia. A great deal of good comes from these individual programs, but an integrated, overall program would be much greater than the sum of its parts.

The Philadelphia Model

Several years ago, I was asked to testify before the Philadelphia Board of Education on the value of having school-based counseling centers address sexuality issues in high schools. Part of the center's responsibility would be distributing condoms to students who requested them. Of the 40 high schools in the city, currently 10 have funded programs for sexual advice, counseling, and condoms. There are political and legal efforts to stop this activity, but it continues to grow and has become an accepted activity among students. Unfortunately, funds are insufficient to cover all 40 high schools and the middle schools.

At the same time sexuality issues were being addressed, the school board also wanted to find a way to resolve the issue of escalating violence in the schools. Because I had become friends with several members of the school administration through my involvement in addressing the sexuality issues and because I was the director of a center for the study of violence, I was invited to participate. In the ensuing months, four task forces were put in place, and the result was a report that detailed some of the things the school district could do. This report became the basis for much of the work we have done in the past 2 years, including the Adopt-a-School Program.

Adopt-a-School

The concept of Adopt-a-School has been used successfully in a number of schools over the past several years. The idea is for a local hospital or church to adopt a school and provide the school with services and essentials the schools cannot otherwise afford. In Philadelphia, we evolved this idea of recruiting physicians to volunteer their services to a specific school. This came about because school personnel felt efforts should be made to help teachers with the human sexuality curriculum, particularly health and physical education teachers, nurses, school psychologists, and guidance counselors. A steering committee was established by myself and the superintendent of schools to encourage community support and to involve sex education experts from around the city.

The committee decided that the first course of action was to hold an in-service training program for teachers and other school personnel. The training included role-playing and other important techniques that the teachers could use with their students. Without going into great detail, it is sufficient to say that the program was not a great success. We learned that talking at teachers and developing small-group educational projects over a 2-day period was not what the teachers wanted. They wanted direct information about how to behave, what to say, and what techniques to use to make their lives easier.

This led to the development of the Adopt-a-School concept. The job of the steering committee was to recruit physicians who were willing to commit themselves to schools. Currently, we have 53 volunteer physicians on board working in 53 different schools. The assignments are made by the school district; the principal of the assigned school is informed early on and becomes an active participant. The result is that these 53 schools now have a physician they can call a member of their faculty.

All specialties, not just psychiatry, have been recruited. The physicians are instructed first to get together with the principal of the school they are assigned to and develop a course of action. For example, a pediatrician was asked to conduct all the physicals required of students going out for sports teams; an obstetrician taught health classes about sex and sexuality; and a pediatrician, working in an elementary school, was asked to look for potentially serious health or immunization problems, as well as identify any disturbed children.

The goal—to have 257 physicians, one for each school—is still a long way off. I am surprised, and saddened, that in a city with close to 10,000 physicians, it has been so difficult to get volunteers.

Time-Out Room

Before we implemented the volunteer program I have described, the steering committee thought it should be tested for 1 year in one school in the district. The committee suggested that I go into a school—the Pierce Middle School—and see if the idea, which seemed so promising, would work. Thus began my 3-year involvement with Pierce.

Pierce has an enrollment of about 600 students; all are African American and live in very difficult and dangerous neighborhoods. The school's faculty members are 70% African

Americans. I went into Pierce knowing that the success of the program depended on the support of the principal, Mary Randall, who turned out to be a very strong and caring woman who welcomed me into her school and offered me the opportunity to work with her.

In explaining what we did at Pierce, I do not go into great detail on tangential issues but instead discuss one program that has grown and evolved and that I think ultimately will be in the best interest of the Pierce community.

One of the first things Principal Randall asked me to help out with was the school's "time-out" room. This was the place children were sent, for 1, 2, or 3 days, when they were too bad to stay in the classroom and too good to be suspended. The room generally had between 5 and 15 students, and teachers were assigned to monitor the room on a rotating basis. The first thing I did was spend some time sitting in the time-out room, observing what went on. Not much went on. The room was a drab, dark, and cold place. The children sat in rows doing busy work, with the teacher uninvolved and set apart from the students. "What is this place like?" I asked the students. "Jail," was the answer I got from everyone.

When they said jail, they were not talking about the jail they saw on television or in the movies. They were talking about real jail, something they knew a great deal about. Members of their family or community had all spent time in jail. This was a rather chilling thought. Even worse, when I asked who knew someone who had a gun, every hand went up. Growing up, and even today, I do not know a single person who owns a gun.

After observing the time-out room, I went back to Ms. Randall and suggested that we try to make the room less punitive. These children grew up in an environment of punishment, and heaping more punishment on them was not productive. Before we could go about changing the time-out room, first we had to change the role of the teachers. We developed some in-service training to communicate to the teachers the need for and benefit of making the time-out room less punitive and more supportive to give the children an opportunity to learn to communicate and to deal with issues related to values. A list of 50–75 stimulus words (e.g., love, respect, responsibility, hate, anger, murder) was developed to get students to communicate with one another and the teachers. We found that this was a relatively easy task, particularly if the children, ages 11–14 years, were involved with teachers they trusted.

The teachers were generally enthusiastic and interested in the project, with the exception of one teacher, who was frightened by the idea of the children getting out of control, in addition to being overwhelmed by the concept of such close interaction with the students. He was removed from the project.

One month after we implemented the changes in the time-out room, I visited Pierce. I met with various faculty groups and students to get a sense of how the program was progressing. The biggest complaint was that "the kids liked it so much there they never wanted to leave." I foolishly thought that the job was over and that I had accomplished my goal. But new problems quickly arose.

Because students were asked to do more than keep quiet and do busy work while they were in the time-out room, those children who were most difficult and incorrigible disrupted the learning efforts we were trying to put in place for the other students, which was the reason these children were sent to the time-out room in the first place. The teachers began to feel, and rightly so, that all their efforts were in vain because they again saw their plans disrupted by one or two unruly students.

Nathan Marx, the school counselor, oversaw the program on a day-to-day basis. A dedicated and patient man who realized that nothing difficult happens easily, he, along with the principal and assistant principal, supported the effort to make the new time-out room concept work. The teachers were mixed in their conviction that rehabilitation was a worthwhile idea, and they were also convinced that crimes needed to be punished.

At the end of a year, Ms. Randall proposed to scrap the entire concept in favor of an alternative plan I fully supported. The new plan was to change the time-out room from a 1-, 2-, or 3-day stay into one in which students would be evaluated and assigned to an alternative learning center for no less than a month, and in some cases, for up to a full school year. The idea was to see if we could, through the use of smaller classrooms and teachers trained to handle the emotional and social issues of the students, correct the children's behavior through individualized and small-group teaching and eventually return them to their regular classroom. They could be mainstreamed back into their classes all at once or slowly reintegrated one or two classes at a time. Through modeling that would teach students a better understanding of their role, we hoped students would be better prepared to learn.

In the summer of 1994, Pierce's administrators and teachers were brought together for a full day of in-service training that dealt with the nuts and bolts of implementing this new idea. Plus, they were given a forum to work through some of the issues they thought would be problematic. We also stressed that this new program would involve the entire faculty because this new program would be harder for students to get into. Borderline students, who were once sent to the time-out room for a day or two, would remain in their regular classrooms to enable the hard-core problem children to be dealt with in a less crowded environment that provided them with more one-on-one and small-group settings. Therefore, even the teachers who were not directly involved in teaching the most difficult and disturbed students would still be impacted by the program and needed to understand and support its goals for it to be successful.

Although it still remains to be seen how this new concept will unfold, I am convinced that we are gradually finding the right path and are on to something. Based on my intervention and the cooperation of the administration and teachers, with no extra funding, this is a perfect example of the "intrusion" of a single person on the scene through the Adopt-a-School program.

The hope that this could happen in all 257 schools in Philadelphia remains alive. In fact, it is my dream that we would go even farther and develop an integrated system for the delivery of services in every school that would offer a full range of mental health services, with a special emphasis on intervention in the six epidemics I have identified. Intervention by community physicians in the schools would continue to grow, not as isolated islands of assistance but through a central plan and enthusiastic commitment to meet the needs of our children.

Youth Homicide Committee

I am the chair of a committee of the Philadelphia Health Department known as the Youth Homicide Committee. There are a number of youth fatality committees across the country, but, to my knowledge, our committee, which deals only with homicide, is unique. The committee includes members of the police department, the Department of Human Services, the health department, the school district, the district attorney's office, the probation department, the medical examiner's office, and a number of community agencies. The group meets monthly to review the murders of children, which, unbelievably, number about 15–20 per month.

It became apparent in Philadelphia that a lack of communication between agencies contributed to the number of murders. For example, two children escaped from a delinquency center they were confined to. No one went after them or notified anyone that they had escaped. The two returned home and went back to their neighborhood school. Within a few months, one had been murdered and the other had committed murder.

In the 1993–1994 school year, the city's security department had more than 10,000 incidents of violence in the schools, with approximately 2,500 arrests.

In response to the problem and the lack of communication between different agencies and departments, we began to develop a plan that would attempt to increase the communication among all the different agencies. Just as importantly, in the six regions of the school district, and within those districts on a school-by-school basis, we began to identify children at risk, who had demonstrated problems. For example, we wanted to find a way to connect all the information gathered by the schools, the police, the courts and probation officers, and the city's various health and human services agencies. Some of these children have serious police records that date back to when they were age 10 or 11 years. Using information developed by the school's security force, we identified certain triggers that would identify the children most prone to commit a violent act or be the victim of a violent act. Truancy was one of the easiest triggers to identify and also one of the easiest to monitor. Other triggers are carrying a weapon or beeper to school, fighting with other students or hitting teachers, disorderly conduct, and psychotic behavior. We need to identify the high-risk children and then, through a centralized effort, make available to them the resources and community support that would help them and their families.

The draft plan we developed is as follows.

Proposal

Each school must identify all personnel who are involved in addressing problems of violence and delinquency. Minimally, the disciplinarian (often the assistant principal) and the security officer will work together in identifying, reporting, and collaborating with a regional team. The ideal school committee may consist of the assistant principal, security officer, school nurse, school counselor, and one or two interested teachers.

Each region of the school district will have one (or more) intervention team whose membership will reflect, as closely as possible, the membership of the Youth Homicide Committee. The team, at least, should be representative of the following:

- Schools (region or subregion)
- Police department
- Department of Human Services
- Probation department
- Judicial system (district attorney's office and representatives from the courts)
- Community-based organizations

- Fire department
- Parents (regional parent-teacher associations)
- Students (this is debatable)

In addition, each team will have officially designated health and mental health consultants. Other consultants or agency representatives (e.g., Philadelphia Housing Authority) will be brought in as needed.

An unpublished report (1994) of the Philadelphia Youth Fatality Review Team indicates that members of the intervention team participate in response to an agency mandate, a professional responsibility, and a commitment to the health, safety, and well-being of youth.

For the purposes of this project, the high schools will be in the same cluster as their feeder elementary and middle schools. Students will be referred to the regional team by the school committee if they are involved in any of the following abnormal behaviors:

- Assaults
- Arson and malicious fire incidents
- Alcohol and drug offenses
- Morals offenses (rape, indecent assault, indecent exposure)
- Robbery, theft, burglary
- Vandalism (personal or school property)
- Weapons offenses (carrying or using a gun against another person)
- Extortion
- Truancy
- Disorderly conduct
- Domestic violence
- Child abuse (victim)

Each team member would share information on the referred student to create interventions that would prevent the student's situation from escalating. This process was adopted by the Youth Homicide Committee, and all team members maintain the con-

fidentiality of the information. The routine and systematic review of the high-risk behavior of youths, coupled with the sharing of confidential information among agencies and individuals,
may serve as a better foundation for clarifying risk factors contributing to preventable deaths among our youths.

The referral team will assess each child and triage the child
to a public or private city or community agency or agencies to
ensure proper care and follow-up.

In addition to and in conjunction with the work of the Youth
Homicide Committee and the draft plan I have detailed, members of the central administration of the school district and the
Health Committee of the Board of Education are working on a
similar plan. We are working to combine the two plans and implement a citywide antiviolence program. The light at the end
of the tunnel is the vision of changing children's lives and values
and reducing violence and murder.

The Future

Clearly, there are a variety of approaches and systems that can
be developed. A true mental health facility in a school setting
should include (in addition to evaluation) outpatient therapy
with individual, group, and family counseling. We could even
extend it a step further and develop partial hospitals within
schools that would serve as alternative classroom settings, with
students remaining here for as long as an entire school year. The
concept of intensive case management is truly important if we
hope to solve the problems of individuals and families. My involvement with the school district of Philadelphia came from my
belief that we must begin to consider primary prevention care
to stop the onslaught of violence our children (particularly those
in the inner cities) face. To eliminate many of the problems we
see today before they have a chance to develop, we must begin
by increasing parenting education (which is a topic that would
take me an entire chapter to address properly). Because of an

192 Managing Care, Not Dollars

epidemic of poor parenting, which in turn leads to physical, sexual, mental, and psychological abuse of children and fosters an environment that breeds violence, schools are forced to take on the roles parents traditionally fulfilled and are kept from their primary responsibility: education.

The growth and development of its children is one of the primary ways to judge the success of a society. We are falling short, and psychiatrists must lead the charge to turn things around. It is our duty and responsibility to understand the problems and work to find solutions. The children who need the most help are the ones least likely to come to our offices. Therefore, we must go to them.

In this nation's public schools, 65% of the children live below the poverty line. The successful growth and development of all children, particularly those who grow up in depressed areas filled with violence and destruction, make the development of full-service schools essential. Psychiatrists need to refocus their attention and be leaders in the development of full-service schools. We can address the problems faced by children in terms of planning, fund-raising, development, and systems development, which includes supervision and administration.

In this chapter, I have tried to demonstrate ways for others to enter the school district as helpers, not leaders, and bring their ideas and talents to a population that desperately needs them. The goal is to overcome the difficulties of acceptance and funding and develop a cooperation between public health and public education in every community in the United States. Providing mental health services throughout our schools is a necessity.

References

Comer JP: School Power. New York, Free Press, 1980
Dryfoos JG: Full-Service Schools. San Francisco, CA, Jossey-Bass, 1994

13 The Elderly Patient

Robert P. Roca, M.D., M.P.H.

Because the elderly who are mentally ill require a well-linked, comprehensive array of services to meet their complex needs, they benefit greatly from a highly integrated continuum of care. Their particular blend of problems, however, calls on the continuum to include services that other groups of patients do not regularly require. The most prevalent condition—dementia—is unusual in nongeriatric populations and demands highly specialized therapeutic, supportive, and residential programming. Even conditions that occur frequently in younger mentally ill populations (e.g., schizophrenia, alcoholism) must be managed differently in the elderly. Therefore, the continuum of care must be sufficiently flexible to "adjust for age."

In this chapter, I present the stories of patients who enter the system at different points and follow different trajectories through the continuum. I then describe 1) the five most important conditions that must be managed within the continuum, emphasizing those aspects of the conditions that have implications for the organization of services; 2) four general factors that influence the design of the psychogeriatric continuum; 3) one vision of the ideal service system; and 4) the approximation of

193

that vision that is taking shape at one institution. In the end, it will be clear that serving this population requires extensive networking among providers both inside and outside of the traditional boundaries of mental health.

Five Stories

The following case studies demonstrate several different pathways through the psychogeriatric continuum of care. After each story is a brief discussion of its salient features.

∎ CASE 1

Mrs. G, 75 years old, fainted while sitting on a pier and fell into shallow water. Her son rescued her, and she was admitted to a general hospital for evaluation. During her medical workup, the physician uncovered a history of "panic attacks" and requested psychiatric consultation. The psychiatrist found that her blood alcohol concentration at the time of hospital admission was 200 mg/dL, indicating significant alcohol intoxication. When presented with this information, she acknowledged that she had been drinking heavily ever since her husband had begun showing signs of possible Alzheimer's disease. She had cared for his demented sister for several years before her death and now feared that she would be faced with even more overwhelming burdens as her husband's caregiver. Compounding her distress was embarrassment about his declining capacities, leading her to hide his problems from others and thereby depriving herself of help from family members and close friends. Alcohol intoxication provided her with brief periods of respite from her duties and worries.

She underwent medical detoxification while in the hospital and had no further panic attacks. On discharge, she rejected residential alcohol rehabilitation and declined to participate in Alcoholics Anonymous, but she made a commitment to total abstinence and expressed a willingness to see the consulting psychiatrist as an outpatient and to take disulfiram (Antabuse).

Outpatient treatment focused on the maintenance of sobriety and on constructive planning regarding her husband's dementia. She took him for medical evaluation, which confirmed the presence of probable Alzheimer's disease, and she began to speak more openly about his impairment with family members, many of whom came forward with offers of assistance. She engaged the services of a housekeeper and joined a support group sponsored by the Alzheimer's Association. As his functional capacity declined, she enrolled him in a medical day program to provide him with structured activity and to afford her respite from her caregiving duties. When he subsequently developed urinary incontinence and began wandering out of the house at night, she decided to place him in a long-term care facility in their community. Although she felt sad about his condition, she did not feel overwhelmed and was able to maintain her sobriety.

This case illustrates the role of the general hospital as a point of entry into the psychogeriatric continuum of care. Mrs. G's general physician was the case finder, and the general hospital (or consultation-liaison) psychiatrist was the primary therapist and case manager. Mrs. G made use of homemaker services, medical day care, a peer support program, and ultimately long-term residential care in a nursing facility. Although many of the providers and services in this case were not formal mental health providers or services, they played a critical role in Mrs. G's mental health outcome. The psychogeriatric continuum must be integrally linked with just such an array of services and providers.

■ CASES 2 AND 3

Dr. S arrived at the nursing home for his routine weekly rounds. The medical director requested that he see Mrs. A and Mr. B. Mrs. A was a demented but highly mobile 98-year-old woman who regularly wandered out of the building and into the street. She had no psychiatric history. Her dementia had first become apparent 6 years earlier, and the workup yielded a diagnosis of probable Alzheimer's disease. She was always cheerful and enjoyed holding a stuffed animal as though it were her child. She had no signs of persecutory delusions or hallucinations. Her Mini-Mental State Examination score was 10/30. Inspection of her immediate environment revealed that her room was adjacent to a door leading outside the building. The nurses confirmed that she often sat outside her room next to the door and watched people go in and out of the building. It appeared that she was simply following them out the door or perhaps imitating them. The psychiatrist suggested that they relocate her down the hall so that she would not be in proximity to the door. He recommended no psychotropic medications.

Mr. B was a vigorous, demented 83-year-old man who was referred because he was punching and grabbing nursing staff as they tried to provide routine care. He had no history of psychiatric illness but had a 4-year history of worsening cognitive impairment. His placement in the nursing home had been precipitated by episodes of assaultiveness directed against his caregivers.

On examination, he was restless and poorly cooperative. He repeated that he wanted to go home and became progressively more angry as he reiterated this wish. He showed generalized suspiciousness but did not have organized delusions. He was disoriented to place and time. Because of the patient's suspiciousness and recent assaultiveness, the psychiatrist recommended a neuroleptic in a low dose.

Three days later, the psychiatrist received a call from the director of nursing. Mrs. A was much better. She had been relocated within the facility and was no longer leaving the building. (She had incidentally become incontinent of urine because she did not yet know the location of the bathroom in her new room.) In contrast, Mr. B was worse. He slept briefly after receiving the medication but was quite irritable when fully awake. Earlier that day, he had grabbed a nurse by the throat, and the efforts of several staff members were needed to free her. This outburst demonstrated that he could not safely be treated in the nursing home, and he was transferred to a psychogeriatric inpatient unit where the consulting psychiatrist had attending privileges.

While on the unit, his neuroleptic dosage was adjusted, and the nursing staff learned how to redirect him without provoking angry responses. Seven days after admission, the directors of nursing and of social work visited the inpatient unit and discussed the patient's progress and status with his psychiatrist and the charge nurse. Five days later, he returned to the nursing home uneventfully. His neuroleptic dosage was subsequently reduced, and he has had no further aggressive outbursts.

These cases illustrate the role of the psychiatrist in the nursing home and the value of a close liaison between the nursing home and the psychogeriatric inpatient unit in the management of difficult patients, particularly those who are assaultive. In nursing home consultation work, the psychiatrist may function independently or may collaborate with a social worker or nurse.

▌ CASE 4

Ms. H was an 80-year-old woman with a long history of schizophrenia. She had never married and now lived by herself in public housing for the elderly. She had recently been treated on an inpatient psychiatric unit for an acute psychotic exacerbation and was scheduled to go to the outpatient clinic for follow-up. She never made it to the clinic, however, because she was afraid to go out of the building. She gradually ran out of her antipsychotic medications and became progressively more symptomatic.

The building management noticed her deterioration and requested an on-site evaluation by the mobile psychogeriatric consultation team. The team nurse interviewed Ms. H in her home and confirmed the presence of delusions and hallucinations. The patient had no insight into her need for care but was willing to have the nurse return. The team psychiatrist accompanied the nurse on a subsequent visit, performed a focused diagnostic interview, and prescribed an antipsychotic medication. The nurse returned at least weekly thereafter to reevaluate Ms. H and to monitor the effects of treatment. As she improved, she expressed a willingness to go to the outpatient clinic to receive ongoing care. The team nurse helped her to secure transportation to these appointments and then checked on her monthly to confirm that she was stable and in treatment.

In this case, it was critical to have a nonprofessional case finder (i.e., the housing manager) available to make the referral and a mobile team of professionals to provide on-site evaluation and treatment. Mentally ill elderly persons who are isolated or who lack interested relatives usually are unidentified and untreated until severe illness or catastrophe (e.g., house fire) ensues. Nonprofessionals can be effective sources of psychogeriatric referral in congregate housing as well as in the community at large. The capacity to bring evaluation and treatment services to the patient is critical to the success of efforts to treat the mentally ill elderly who are most in need of care. Psychiatric home health nursing and multidisciplinary mobile treatment teams serve this purpose.

▌ CASE 5

Mrs. R was a 75-year-old woman with bipolar disorder and a history of frequent, lengthy hospitalizations for manic episodes. She lived with her daughter-in-law and her young grandson. When well, she was quiet and helpful with housework. When manic, she was boisterously cheerful, impulsive, intrusive, disorganized, and sleepless. Her family would bring her to the emergency room and refuse to allow her to return home until her mania had completely resolved; this typically took at least 3 months. Recently her family notified her psychiatrist early in the course of a typical manic relapse. Because she was not yet floridly symptomatic and was unwilling to come to the office several times a week for close monitoring, arrangements were made for psychiatric home health nursing visits. The home health nurse performed an assessment, contacted the referring psychiatrist, and collaborated with him on a treatment plan involving close medication monitoring and meticulous efforts to support the family. The nurse herself visited twice weekly and also arranged for a home health aide to assist the patient with personal care and related activities several times a week. Over the course of 3 months, the patient gradually improved, and hospitalization never became necessary.

The ability of the nurse-psychiatrist team to go into the community to treat the patient and support the family on site was critical to this outcome.

Five Common Conditions

The clinical vignettes illustrate some of the problems and needs that must be addressed by the psychogeriatric continuum of care. Many of these follow directly from the characteristics of the conditions that are most prevalent in this population.

Dementia

Dementia is a syndrome of cognitive decline in clear consciousness. It affects at least 5% of persons older than age 65 years and 20% of persons older than age 80 years, making it one of the most common psychiatric disorders of late life. Because the age group at highest risk (the "old-old") is also the most rapidly growing segment of the population, dementia will be a public health problem of increasing importance over the next several decades.

Alzheimer's disease is the most common cause of dementia in the United States, accounting for at least half of cases. Most of the remainder are due to cerebrovascular disease or admixtures of cerebrovascular disease and Alzheimer's disease. These conditions are neither curable nor reversible, but there are several opportunities for useful intervention. Because cognitive functioning in demented patients is exquisitely sensitive to the effects of medical illness (e.g., pneumonia, urinary tract infections) and polypharmacy, good general medical care is a vital component of treatment. In addition, about one-third of patients with Alzheimer's disease may show modest, temporary improvement in cognitive functioning in response to tacrine (Cognex), a newly approved drug that enhances central cholinergic neurotransmission. Furthermore, because more than two-thirds of demented patients exhibit troublesome "noncognitive" behavioral and psychiatric symptoms (e.g., aggressiveness, wandering, delusions, hallucinations, "agitation"), most demented patients benefit from behavioral and/or pharmacological treatment by mental health professionals who are experienced in the management of these problems. Such management usually involves measures to support the caregiver as well as to treat the patient. Ultimately, most demented persons require 24-hour nursing care at home or in a long-term care facility.

Dementia care thus calls for a system that provides ready access to general medical care as well as psychogeriatric consultation, medical day care, respite care, social work, home care, and long-term nursing services. The nature of the problems and the limitations of the patients often require that care be provided on site, that is, not in offices but in the private homes or nursing facilities where patients reside. The care of these patients will be the most challenging problem facing the psychogeriatric continuum of care in the decades to come.

Delirium

It is critical to distinguish dementia from delirium—a state of global cognitive impairment associated with disturbances in consciousness and attention. Delirium is the mental and behavioral manifestation of acute physical illness or drug toxicity and usually resolves when the underlying medical problem is effectively treated. Its prognosis and treatment are thus very different from those of dementia, even though the clinical appearance of delirium and dementia may be superficially similar. The consultation-liaison or general hospital psychiatrist is in the best position to make the diagnosis and to guide his or her physician colleagues in the evaluation and management of this condition.

Major Depression

The core features of major depression include sadness, self-dissatisfaction, and diminished physical and mental vitality. It may be triggered by a particular disappointment or loss or may arise "endogenously" (from within). Recent epidemiological data indicate that major depression is not a necessary concomitant of aging: its prevalence actually *declines* with age. Nonetheless, it constitutes an important public health problem because 3% of the elderly population are currently affected, and the absolute numbers of depressed elderly persons will continue to grow as our national demography shifts in the years to come.

Although the principal manifestations of major depression do not vary significantly with age, elderly depressive persons are more likely than younger patients to have prominent somatic symptoms, delusions of poverty, successful suicide attempts, and reversible deficits in performance on tests of cognitive function. One of the most important therapeutic implications of major depression in general is a high probability of response to antidepressant medications. It is likely that this favorable prognosis applies to elderly depressive patients as well as younger ones, even though the elderly are underrepresented in most studies of antidepressant efficacy and often experience life stresses (e.g., acute and chronic medical illnesses) that reduce the chances of an optimal outcome. Furthermore, they are often less tolerant of antidepressant side effects than younger persons and therefore must be monitored very closely to ensure both compliance and safety as adequate dosages are achieved.

Schizophrenia and Delusional Disorders

DSM-III (American Psychiatric Association 1980) did not permit the diagnosis of schizophrenia in cases in which the age at onset exceeds 45 years. It is now recognized that this condition may begin in late life, particularly among women. Delusional disorders may also begin after age 45. Both conditions respond to antipsychotic medications and are therefore important to detect and treat. Two factors militate against their detection. First, persons with these disorders often live solitary lives, at least partly as a result of persecutory delusions, and almost never come forward voluntarily for treatment. Second, they may be misdiagnosed as demented when they finally do come to attention. These facts require that the psychogeriatric continuum of care include the capacity for community-based case finding and referral as well as expert diagnostic evaluation.

Alcoholism and Prescription Drug Abuse

Although the rates of substance abuse decline with age, alcoholism and prescription drug abuse do occur among the elderly. In most instances, the habits of abuse are of long standing; however, about one-third of problematic elderly drinkers begin drinking heavily in late life, often in response to age-specific social factors (see case 1). Although the fundamental principles of treatment (e.g., the goal of total abstinence) are indifferent to age, the elderly tend to require more intensive monitoring during detoxification, slower detoxification, and special sensitivity to age-specific issues in educational and rehabilitative programming.

Four Factors Affecting the Organization of Services

The geriatric continuum of services must be adequate to the task of managing the most prevalent conditions found among the elderly. In addition, the specific design of these services must take into account special developmental, biological, psychological, and social considerations.

Developmental Principle

A critical overarching consideration in the design of services for the elderly is that there is great age-dependent variability among persons termed *elderly*. This means that the problems and needs of the average 65-year-old differ greatly from those of the average 90-year-old. An effective psychogeriatric continuum will reflect this developmental understanding in its array of services.

Biological, Psychological, and Social Factors

The design of services must also take into account a number of age-related biological, psychological, and social factors. Older persons often have dental problems, impairments in sensory function, and chronic medical conditions that usually require medications or other forms of corrective intervention. Even those without serious comorbid medical conditions need to be treated with special care because of age-specific biological vulnerabilities such as changes in drug pharmacokinetics. The psychogeriatric continuum of care should be staffed by clinicians who have training in geriatric medicine and the biology of aging.

Even nondemented elderly persons tend to experience age-related decrements in performance on tests of memory and other cognitive and psychomotor functions. These changes affect many domains of their lives and may compromise their ability to keep appointments, adhere to medication schedules, and cooperate with other aspects of their medical care. Elderly mentally ill persons are additionally burdened by psychiatric symptoms that frequently compound their difficulty maneuvering through the general health care system. For this reason, they benefit greatly from the willingness of their mental health providers to help coordinate their general health care.

Most elderly persons have fixed incomes and struggle to cover the rising costs of medications and other expensive necessities. It is often impossible or unsafe for them to drive and costly or otherwise unacceptable for them to use other means of transportation, leaving them isolated and unable to make scheduled appointments. They often require live-in caregivers who may or may not be competent and who, in any case, usually need support in their own right. The ideal geriatric continuum will recognize and respond to all of these social needs.

Characteristics of the Ideal System

What are the implications of all these considerations for a service system? The ideal system would be responsive to the unique epidemiology of mental disorders among the elderly and would take into account the developmental, biological, psychological, and social factors already mentioned. A system developed in response to all these considerations would include three broad categories of services: 1) age-sensitive diagnostic, therapeutic, and rehabilitative services for patients; 2) programs to support caregivers; and 3) programs to case-find (i.e., to identify those in need of care who might not otherwise come to attention).

Services for Patients

Services for psychogeriatric patients need to be *appropriately intensive.* Most patients do not need inpatient care; however, patients who are assaultive, suicidal, acting on hallucinations, or unresponsive to less restrictive interventions need to be hospitalized, and this is best done on an inpatient unit specially adapted to their needs. Some patients are severely disabled by affective disorders or anxiety disorders but have stable home environments and do not need around-the-clock nursing; these persons are excellent candidates for day or partial hospital programs. Patients who are less severely disabled, especially those who are beginning to show improvement in response to treatment, are adequately served by office-based care. An ideal system of care would offer all these components and would allow for the treatment of patients by the same clinicians at different levels of care.

Services need to be *highly accessible.* Because many patients cannot or will not leave their living environments to receive care, it is often necessary to make services available to patients where they live. This means that nursing home patients should be able to receive care on-site and that community-dwelling elderly with mobility and/or transportation difficulties should be seen at home or transported to the place of service.

Services must be *multidisciplinary.* In particular, general medical services must be closely integrated with mental health services to help address general medical comorbidity and polypharmacy. Other important services include physical therapy, speech and occupational therapy, social work, pharmacy, dentistry, and personal care.

Services must be *well coordinated.* This requires that the services be well linked to one another and that one clinician or team of clinicians take comprehensive responsibility for the management of the case. The goal of such case management is to ensure that needs are not overlooked and that services are delivered in the most efficient way.

Finally, the services must be *age sensitive.* They should be generally adapted to the needs of the elderly and also reflect the developmental understanding that the needs of the average 65-year-old require a different response than the needs of the average 90-year-old.

Programs for Caregivers

Caregivers have high rates of anxiety and depression, poor general health status, and lots of distress related to the day-to-day demands of caregiving. For these reasons, our systems need to provide caregivers with resources for respite, education, and peer support.

Respite services provide relief from care responsibilities during the day or overnight for variable periods of time. Medical day services (i.e., medical day care programs) offer individualized programs of treatment and rehabilitation, as well as social and leisure activities, for participants with a wide variety of impair-

ments while providing respite for working and/or weary caregivers during daylight hours. Such programs are generally available up to 5 days a week. The length of stay is unlimited. A
number of long-term care (i.e., nursing home) facilities provide
around-the-clock care on a short-term basis to allow caregivers
extended periods of overnight relief. When in-home respite is
most appropriate or acceptable, companions and home health
aides may provide company, supervision, help with personal
care, and other forms of assistance without dislocation or disruption. Although it is usually impractical for such services to be
operated directly by mental health providers, the geriatric mental health continuum of care should at least be closely linked
with providers of adult day, nursing home, and personal care so
that a range of respite services can be offered to the families of
mentally ill elderly persons.

Most caregivers desire education from professionals about
diagnosis, treatment, and prognosis. All clinicians should have
access to problem-specific written materials that address these
topics and may be distributed to caregivers and other interested
parties. Educational videotapes can be prepared or purchased
and then lent to caregivers. Lectures and seminars may be offered at health care facilities or in the community.

Caregivers often benefit greatly from opportunities to hear
how others have managed their caregiving responsibilities. Peer
support groups sponsored by the Alliance for the Mentally Ill or
the Alzheimer's Association may be great sources of practical
assistance and moral support. The geriatric continuum should
provide meeting space for such groups and should encourage
caregivers to participate.

Case Finding

Elderly persons with interested families generally make their
way into the system of care. On the other hand, those who are
extremely isolated and without "intimate advocates" rarely present themselves for care and may come to attention only when
gravely ill or the victims of catastrophe. To identify these persons

earlier, the psychogeriatric continuum must have the capacity for case finding. This capability is strongly enhanced by the development of community education programs that teach non-professionals to recognize the signs of serious mental illness and to report their observations to a responsible body. An excellent model is the Gatekeeper program of the Spokane Mental Health Center in Washington. Conceived by Ray Raschko, director of elderly services, the Gatekeeper program trains bank tellers, postal workers, meter readers, telephone operators, and similar community-based workers to identify signs of mental illness in their clients and customers (e.g., extreme confusion, deteriorating self-care) and encourages them to refer such persons for in-home evaluation by a mobile team from the mental health center. This program has been well accepted and effective. A similar approach, adapted to its special setting, has been utilized effectively by Psychogeriatric Assessment and Treatment in City Housing (PATCH), a program of on-site psychogeriatric assessment and treatment for elderly residents of public housing in Baltimore, Maryland.

Geriatric Services at Sheppard Pratt (Baltimore, Maryland)

The creation of a comprehensive system is an ambitious task, requiring the linkage of diverse services, many of which do not fall within the traditional boundaries of mental health. For this reason, the creation of such a system is beyond the capacity of most mental health providers acting independently. The practical solution is to act collaboratively, to build a network of relationships among diverse providers, forming a multipolar continuum of care that offers comprehensive services to a regional community of need.

An essential component in the creation of such a system is "internal networking," ensuring smooth transitions between levels of care within the base institution. An equally important component is *external* networking, linking with outside providers and agencies to enhance the comprehensiveness of the services available to the patients and caregivers served by the continuum. This has been the approach taken by the Sheppard Pratt Health System. The first move was to link together existing on-campus geriatric programs. This was accomplished when the health system was reorganized along "service lines" in 1992 and two preexisting programs—psychogeriatric inpatient unit and geriatric day (partial) hospital—came under the overall directorship of the Geriatric Service Line. At that point, it became clear that the health system needed to enhance its capacity to do office-based outpatient psychogeriatric evaluation and treatment. The geriatric outpatient program was thus expanded and staffed with clinicians who were already working on the inpatient unit or in the day hospital so that patients moving among levels of care within the health system could continue to receive care from the same clinicians. This triad of services—psychogeriatric inpatient unit, geriatric day hospital, geriatric outpatient services—made up the on-campus core of the psychogeriatric continuum of care.

These on-campus programs had the capacity to serve many patients. Many remained out of reach, however, particularly nursing home residents and persons who were unable or unwilling to leave home. Thus, the obvious next step was to move off campus and deliver care on site. As we contemplated this move, it became clear that we would need to collaborate closely with other agencies and providers in both the private and public sectors. One of the first initiatives was to develop a program of service to local nursing homes and life-care communities. Over a period of months, we developed agreements with several local facilities to provide on-site psychiatric evaluation and treatment. This work was funded by fee-for-service collections, supplemented by a "retainer" paid by the facility to cover administrative expenses, informal consultation to staff, in-service education, and other nonreimbursable activities. The clinicians staffing this activity also worked in the day hospital or on the inpatient unit and thus could continue to care for patients who required treatment in more intensive on-campus settings. We also collaborated with public sector agencies to help provide home-based psychiatric services to mentally ill elderly residing in several local catchment areas.

These diverse activities were all within our expertise as a mental health system. We had little direct experience providing certain other essential services, however, and in these areas we relied on the capabilities of our collaborators, especially acute general hospitals, nursing homes, adult medical day care programs, and home health agencies. Through our relationships with these providers, our patients and their caregivers could be offered respite, home health care, and other services that fall outside the traditional boundaries of mental health but are vital to mental health outcomes for the mentally ill elderly and their caregivers.

Conclusion

The vision of the psychogeriatric continuum of care continues to evolve as gaps in services appear and new opportunities for intervention are discovered. This capacity to evolve will be critical in the years ahead. We will need to make adjustments in our systems of care as the elderly grow more numerous and as we learn more about how best to treat their ailments. Geriatric psychiatry is, after all, a new specialty, and there is much to learn. We can already say, however, that care of the mentally ill elderly calls for a diverse, well-coordinated array of variably intensive services—precisely the sort of organization that a continuum of care model can offer. We can say that the particular design of the psychogeriatric continuum must take into account a number of age-specific biological, psychological, and social considerations. In addition, we can say that the system must have the capacity to manage a distinctive epidemiology (e.g., complicated dementias), to operate in nontraditional settings (e.g., nursing homes), and to access modalities (e.g., adult day care services) that are not generally pertinent to nonelderly populations and may not even fall within the usual boundaries of mental health services. To do this requires more than internal coordination of care: it requires external networking, collaborating with providers of other relevant services in an integrated effort to eliminate the gaps in services that could compromise mental health outcomes for patients and families. The ideal system is thus not a mental hospital, a community mental health center, or even a mental health system. It is rather a multiprofessional, multipolar continuum of collaborating health, social, and residential resources—drawn from the public and private sectors—serving a regional community of need.

Reference

American Psychiatric Association: Diagnostic and Statistical Manual of Mental Disorders, 3rd Edition. Washington, DC, American Psychiatric Association, 1980

Additional Readings

Assertive at-home case management for impaired elderly persons: elderly services program, Spokane (Washington) Community Mental Health Center. Hospital and Community Psychiatry 39:1201–1202, 1988

Baltes P: The aging mind: potential and limits. Gerontologist 33:580–594, 1993

Roca RP, Storer DJ, Robbins BM, et al: Psychogeriatric assessment and treatment in urban public housing. Hospital and Community Psychiatry 41:916–920, 1990

Santmyer KS, Roca RP: Geropsychiatry in long-term care: a nurse-centered approach. J Am Geriatr Soc 39:156–159, 1991

III

Planning and
Administering the
Continuum

14 The Economic Case for the Continuum of Care

Ronald D. Geraty, M.D.
Robert J. Fox, J.D.

As recently as the early to mid-1980s, inpatient and office-based outpatient treatment were the only available alternatives in the bifurcated treatment setting frameworks of most behavioral health care environments. The vast majority of health benefit plans were designed so reimbursement for inpatient hospitalization was very heavily favored over payment for treatment provided in outpatient settings. Compared with inpatient benefits, most outpatient psychiatric benefits were restricted and subject to severe coverage and reimbursement limitations.

Under this "benefit-driven" system, financial biases toward inpatient care were fostered, and both patients and providers of care were obliged to heed the dictates of perverse fiscal incentives that drove treatment toward more costly institutional inpa-

213

tient settings. Unfortunately, the benefit-driven framework constricted care delivery into a narrow paradigm that bore only a limited relationship to the primary clinical needs of appropriateness and effectiveness of treatment setting and modality. Ironically, the oddly skewed benefit-driven design failed to attain its primary objective—cost containment.

As costs continued to mount, the focus of the benefit-driven system shifted inward on itself, and more drastic limitations on reimbursement for inpatient care were instituted. Typically, tighter annual limits on reimbursable inpatient days were imposed, and retrospective utilization review was instituted. As with restrictions on outpatient care, benefit limitations were implemented irrespective of their relationship to the best clinical interests of the patient. Although considerable declines in inpatient treatment costs were realized, concerned professionals were becoming disabled in their efforts to promote access to appropriate care in an appropriate setting.

During the 1980s, there was also a widespread introduction and expansion of managed care techniques as applied to the delivery of psychiatric and chemical dependency care. A brief review of that recent history lends insight into the development and management of the continuum of care in the delivery of behavioral treatment to millions of Americans.

The first generation of managed care in psychiatric and chemical dependency treatment delivery could be characterized as one of *managed access.* At this stage, the main focus was on limiting patient access and containing costs through the implementation of benefit coverage limitations and administrative barriers. Under a system in which treatment precertification was the fundamental management technique, primarily nonclinical or nonpsychiatric reviewers placed emphasis on limiting or restricting patient access. Care providers were not included as an active part of the managed care system but mostly were dealt with as outsiders.

The evolution of mental health managed care continued during a second stage of *managed benefits,* which employed utilization review with discounted fee-for-service reimbursement to noncontracted provider networks. The objective was to better control costs through health benefit plan designs that included greater patient out-of-pocket outlays. In this way, emphasis was placed primarily on managing patients' health benefits. Although precertification continued to be a core technique, significant co-pays for plan beneficiaries were introduced as another primary cost-containment method, and overall treatment planning (clinical management) continued to be a secondary consideration. Traditional treatment models were employed. Although providers were somewhat "included" under this approach, their care delivery was still "inspected."

One of the greatest flaws of benefit-driven reimbursement systems and early "managed care" approaches was a vision that failed to look much beyond the inpatient setting. The concentration of energies on cost containment, through inpatient benefit manipulation or utilization management applied almost exclusively to the inpatient milieu, bred a neglect of the clinical goal of serving the full range of individual patient needs. The crucial interrelatedness between the inpatient setting and other points on the continuum of care was basically ignored.

The third evolutionary stage of managed psychiatric care has brought what can truly be termed *managed care*. Quite apart from the previous managed care stages, there has been a shift toward improving access and benefits as a means of reducing costs. The major emphasis of this managed behavioral health care system is the case management of the clinical process. Utilization management of a quality-based, selectively contracted, interdisciplinary provider network has placed greater concentration on treatment planning and quality management, with a focus on the most appropriate care in the most appropriate setting. Case management has become a key means of properly managing patient care throughout the full continuum of care delivery settings. A cost study of this managed behavioral health care approach indicated that cost savings of 30%–40% are regularly achieved (Geraty et al. 1994). With improved provider-case manager collegiality, providers have become an integral part of the clinical management process.

Now managed behavioral health care is progressing into a fourth generation of *managed outcome*. As opposed to earlier stages of managed care, not only are cost savings spotlighted, but also proof of improved treatment quality and outcome is being required. The need for better clinical management is becoming even more acute as the industry, which previously had served mainly beneficiaries under employer-paid benefit plans, is realizing growth opportunities in public programs (e.g., Medicaid, Medicare), which will require the management of more complex patient populations that include greater numbers of seriously and persistently mentally ill individuals, physically disabled, and indigent families with children and adolescents. Additionally, the objectives of improved quality and outcome require "reintegration" and better coordination among primary care providers and the general medical system in recognition of their integral roles in the delivery of behavioral health care.

To meet and surpass fourth-generation market expectations, *integrated behavioral health care systems,* which will manage the entire scope of clinical, financial, and operational functions of the care delivery system, are being created. As part of that process, managed behavioral health care companies are entering into closer partnerships with providers who constitute a full continuum of care, and one result is an overlap in the roles of providers and managed care organizations. Specifically, providers are moving to full risk-sharing roles in the form of per-episode fees and capitation payments. Greater risk assumption by providers requires them to enhance administrative capabilities in finance, actuarial, and information systems as care delivery moves beyond the merely clinical and requires the complex skills necessary to manage financial and operational data in delivering the best quality of care at the lowest possible price at the most appropriate point on the continuum. Optimizing treatment efficacy, while maintaining cost efficiencies, yields the greatest value for each health care dollar spent. Managed behavioral health care continues to incorporate risk-sharing incentives to maximize the potential of the entire continuum to increase value in the delivery of care.

The continuum of care encompasses a range of treatment settings and modalities varying in location and intensity of service. Without a familiarity with managed behavioral health care efficiencies, one might consider the new treatment possibilities of the continuum to be the source of additive costs. However, particularly in light of the past overemphasis on the inpatient treatment setting, the continuum offers lower-cost treatment services (e.g., partial hospitalization, intensive outpatient, home based) that in many cases were previously unavailable. Alternatives to 24-hour hospitalization have proven to contain costs by avoiding unnecessary and expensive inpatient treatment, reducing recidivism, and producing positive outcomes. An analysis of employer-sponsored health benefit plans prepared by the Hay/Huggins Company (1992) provides evidence that the continuum reduces the cost of psychiatric care. It is through the proper management of care delivered within the continuum that cost savings and clinical efficacy can be maximized. The availability of a wider range of treatment choices during the full course of treatment improves the opportunities for delivering more appropriate and, therefore, more effective care. More effective care produces better outcomes, and improved outcomes yield cost benefits in terms of reduced utilization.

The current movement to a broad continuum of care is well evidenced by the private psychiatric hospital industry's attempts to fill the gaps in the continuum. Whereas at one time the service offered by these institutions was almost exclusively inpatient treatment, in 1994 nearly 25% of admissions to surveyed private psychiatric hospitals were for partial hospitalization, outpatient care, and residential treatment (up from only 11% in 1992). Furthermore, the percentage of these hospitals offering partial hospitalization grew from 89% in 1992 to 93% in 1994 (National Association of Psychiatric Health Systems 1995). Studies demonstrate that partial hospitalization can yield savings of as much as 50% when used to shorten length of inpatient stay (Parker and Knoll 1990). Impressive savings have been achieved at all points along the continuum, including specialized approaches such as psychosocial rehabilitation day programs and halfway houses. All appropriate uses of these alternative treatment approaches have delivered care that is at least as effective as hospitalization.

The identified points on the continuum are not distinctly separate, but they indicate levels of care that are interrelated elements of the treatment spectrum (see Figure 14–1). Effective management enables a timely and rational patient flow, as necessary and appropriate, from one treatment point to another as needed during the course of care. In this manner, the delivery of the most appropriate treatment at the right time and place is facilitated; this, in turn, makes possible the delivery of the greatest treatment value.

Individualized case management has been a hallmark technique of managed behavioral health care, and, with the increasing acceptance and deployment of the many treatment options offered by a continuum of care, the case management function becomes even more important. As a given treatment episode progresses, the transition of the patient to less intensive levels

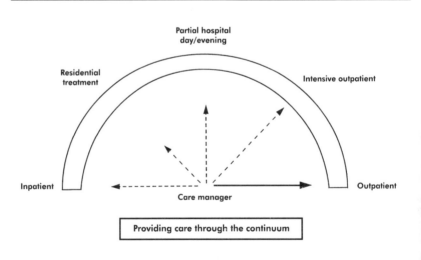

Figure 14–1.   Treatment continuum.

of care, as appropriate, can be facilitated by the case manager. Within an integrated behavioral health care system, featuring centrally available patient information, this movement can be achieved without the traditional duplicative administrative burdens encountered when a patient moves to a new level of care. The integration of information and financial systems creates an operational environment conducive to the efficient use of the continuum. Integrated behavioral health care delivery systems can achieve a higher degree of clinical and cost efficiency when care delivery is not burdened by cumbersome benefit-driven disincentives that hamper the choice of the most appropriate treatment level. As the popularity of indemnity health coverages wanes and care managers and providers more frequently assume full risk for delivery of care under capitation and fee-per-episode arrangements, greater financial incentives toward clinical and cost efficiency are created.

As Table 14–1 shows, offering treatment in a broader range of settings affords the ability not only to reduce total costs, but also to increase the units of service provided to patients. The cost figures and units of service in Table 14–1 are not drawn from any specific behavioral health care program for a particular patient population. Rather, based on the authors' experience, this illustrative model presents general data representing the cost-effectiveness of managed care techniques as compared with more traditional care delivery approaches. Presented in this model are utilization and cost patterns encountered under four different care delivery and reimbursement approaches: indemnity, managed indemnity, managed care, and risk assumption. For cost illustration purposes, Table 14–1 provides anticipated figures for units of service, estimated unit costs, and total costs for a given patient population under the four alternative approaches to reimbursement and care delivery. Figures within the four approaches are broken out according to the example of the commonly utilized treatment settings presented in the table: inpatient, partial hospitalization, intensive outpatient, and outpatient.

As illustrated, under the indemnity and managed indemnity approaches, service delivery is generally restricted to either in-

Table 14-1. Economic case for the continuum

	Indemnity			Managed indemnity			Managed care			Risk assumption		
	Units	Unit cost	Total costs	Units	Unit cost	Total costs	Units	Unit cost	Total costs	Units	Unit cost	Total costs
Inpatient	120	$800	$96.0K	90	$800	$72.0K	40	$500	$20.0K	30	$500	$15.0K
Partial hospital-ization	—	—	—	—	—	—	30	$125	$3.7K	30	$125	$3.7K
Intensive outpatient	—	—	—	—	—	—	—	—	—	30	$70	$2.1K
Outpatient	300	$125	$37.5K	300	$100	$30.0K	400	$80	$32.0K	400	$70	$28.0K
Grand totals	420		$133.5K	390		$102.0K	470		$55.7K	490		$48.8K

patient or outpatient care, with no contemplation of services being delivered in partial hospitalization or intensive outpatient settings. Further, the fee-for-service reimbursement typical of indemnity and managed indemnity approaches serves generally to maintain the number of units of service, unit costs, and total costs at relatively high levels.

In contrast, the range of available treatment settings is expanded under the illustrated managed care (addition of partial hospitalization) and risk assumption (addition of partial hospitalization and intensive outpatient) approaches. These managed approaches to the use of a broader continuum of care serve to reduce unnecessary and inappropriate utilization (units of service) and per-unit costs of expensive inpatient treatment while increasing the number of units of service properly delivered in less intensive partial hospitalization, intensive outpatient, and outpatient settings. In fact, the total number of units of service delivered is increased under the managed care and risk assumption approaches through the appropriate delivery of care along the full continuum. At the same time, unit costs and overall costs are decreased through negotiated reimbursement arrangements with providers.

A brief overview of the four reimbursement and care delivery approaches provides further details of the continuum's economic efficiency.

Within the unmanaged indemnity system, which today represents less than 10% of health coverages in the United States, care delivery is generally limited to either inpatient or outpatient settings. Although the administrative expenses of such a system, as a percentage of total cost of care, are relatively low at 8%–10%, the prohibitive level of overall costs of care have pushed the unmanaged indemnity system to the brink of extinction.

Under managed indemnity approaches, the basic indemnity system remains largely the same, except for certain cursory restraints in the form of utilization review and inpatient benefit limitations. In this environment, although inpatient utilization is reduced somewhat and outpatient costs are decreased, the potentials of a continuum beyond traditional inpatient and out-

patient settings remain largely unexplored. In fact, although total costs are reduced, these savings are achieved only through a
decrease in the total number of units of service delivered to patients. The expense of introducing rudimentary management
controls to the delivery system can raise administrative costs to
the 10%–12% range. Nearly one-third of current benefit coverages can be characterized as managed indemnity.

As illustrated in Table 14–1, established managed care systems generally have served to expand the range of continuum
settings used in the delivery of care. Specifically, partial hospitalization has been an effective alternative to treatment that otherwise would have been provided in more expensive and
restrictive inpatient settings. Additionally, the principles of early
intervention and individualized case management have resulted
in more care being appropriately provided in outpatient settings. Through proper quality management of contracted, interdisciplinary provider networks, significant reductions in service
unit costs in inpatient and outpatient settings have been
achieved, while the total units of delivered care have increased.
In this way, negotiated reimbursement rates, coupled with the
channeling of patients to the most appropriate, least restrictive
treatment setting in a broader continuum, make possible the
delivery of more care to a greater number of patients at a lower
cost. The reduction in inpatient utilization has been particularly
noteworthy in this effort. The added demands of closely managing the delivery of care can result in administrative costs equal-
ing 20%–25% of total cost of care—a price that is well worthwhile
in light of overall cost reductions.

Within emerging risk assumption approaches, by which integrated behavioral health care systems and providers assume
greater accountability for both clinical *and* financial efficiency
of the delivery system, an expanded use of the continuum of care
and more sophisticated management techniques are capable of
reducing costs even further. Again, the movement of patients to
less restrictive, more appropriate levels of care yields the positive aspects of reduced costs and an increase in units of service
delivered. The widespread development of alternative treatment

approaches, such as intensive outpatient programs, improves both clinical efficacy and fiscal efficiency. An enhanced integration of providers with delivery systems that assume financial risk may be able to systematize the proper incentives to deliver care in the most effective and efficient manner (Rofman and Curran 1995). The provision of more clinically effective care decreases overall costs through lower rates of recidivism and repeat episodes (Coursey et al. 1990). This is the essence of behavioral health care value. With a deeper financial stake in the efficacy of treatment, providers achieve value through the optimization of treatment results. The use of the full continuum of care enables care managers and providers to optimize clinical outcomes by more flexibly individualizing the treatment plan to the needs of the patient. The incentives of capitation and fee-per-episode arrangements further ensure that care is delivered when it is medically necessary and appropriate. Although these systems of sophisticated integration of management, clinical, and financial functions require more thorough administrative controls (administrative costs may range up to 25%–30% of total cost of care), the efficiencies attained more than justify the cost elements.

The continuing evolution of reimbursement and care delivery from indemnity to managed indemnity to managed care to risk assumption systems has expanded the loci of treatment beyond traditional inpatient and outpatient settings to a broader care continuum. It is important to note that the continuum of care is not a static construct but is expansive, and developing care delivery systems, particularly for seriously and persistently mentally ill persons within public programs, continues to broaden the scope of available treatment services and settings. Augmenting treatment possibilities enhances access to high-quality care while improving cost-effectiveness (Cole et al. 1994; Reed et al. 1994). A concomitant of improved savings has been a greater focus on professional practices, as Figure 14–2 illustrates. With progress toward more effective and efficient care delivery has come the necessity for providers to adopt more advanced and comprehensive management systems.

Inpatient facilities have accelerated their development of service and information systems that establish important linkages and practice bonds with less costly aftercare and alternative sources of care. Outpatient providers have adjusted to the realities of behavioral health care management. As the breadth of the continuum has grown over the last decade, institutional facilities, group practices, and individual practitioners have encountered considerable administrative challenges in linking with a multitude of reimbursement and clinical management systems used by various payers, care managers, and other providers. Without an efficient integration of clinical, management, and financial functions, the availability of a full continuum of services does not necessarily translate into access to a full spectrum of care. To sustain cost-effectiveness through efficacy of treatment, particularly for seriously mentally ill persons, it is of paramount importance that continuity of care be maintained when patients

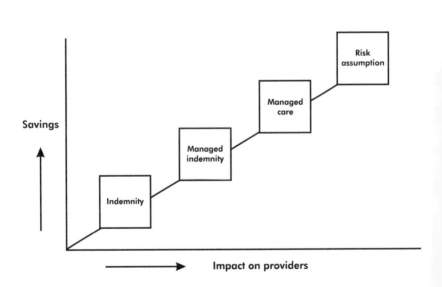

Figure 14-2. Savings and impact on providers.

move from one level of care or treatment setting to another on the continuum.

One of the hallmarks in the success of the managed behavioral health care industry has been the implementation of advanced case management techniques. Individualized case management works to ensure continuity of care and a smooth transition between treatment settings and is generally regarded as the most effective means of maximizing the progress of the patient within the continuum. Moreover, research indicates that case management is successful in reducing overall costs of treatment by ensuring that patients receive appropriate types and levels of service.

To successfully case manage the delivery and promote continuity of effective care in the emerging behavioral health care environment, unprecedented coordination of the activities of all stakeholders in the delivery system will be necessary. The management, processing, and communication of clinical and operational data as part of sophisticated interactions between providers, managers, and payers will be a cornerstone in establishing clinical value. Just as no single provider in the continuum can operate in a solitary fashion, all forces in the world of behavioral health care will require meaningful and efficient information system linkages that promote the clinical interests of patients.

Currently, the health care industry features a maze of primarily uncoordinated clinical, operational, and research information systems with a wide variety of data collection, electronic interchange, and clinical data set configurations. Providing care within this often puzzling, incongruent universe can entail a high level of administrative frustration. The duplication of effort and moment-to-moment adaptation to the idiosyncrasies of incompatible system requirements not only complicate the delivery of care, but also impose additional cost burdens.

Efforts are now under way in the behavioral health care industry to establish data and communication system norms and standards that will bring an acceptable level of uniformity to clinical, management, and financial interactions. Particularly as the degree of interaction among providers at different points on the care continuum increases, the need for such standardization will become even more apparent. Because clinical efficacy is at the heart of cost-effectiveness, the ability to conduct multisystem outcome studies spanning a wide variety of treatment settings and patient populations and to improve the delivery of care on that basis will be crucial to future cost efficiency.

Of course, the architecture of the continuum of care has not been and will not be fixed or unchangeable. Experience and research will provide further insights into the optimal uses of existing resources and will create a foundation from which to explore the deployment of new treatment settings and modalities. Any systemic standardization must therefore allow a flexibility that promotes innovation and creativity in the quest to deliver high-quality, cost-effective care.

To date, the clinical and economic advantages of a versatile continuum of care have fostered continued progress in behavioral health care treatment delivery. More importantly, the continuum will be fertile ground for the even greater achievements of tomorrow.

References

Cole RE, Reed SK, Babigian HM, et al: A mental health capitation program, I: patient outcomes. Hospital and Community Psychiatry 45:1090–1096, 1994

Coursey RD, Ward-Alexander L, Katz B: Cost-effectiveness of providing insurance benefits for posthospital psychiatric halfway house stays. Am Psychol 45:1118–1126, 1990

Geraty R, Bartlett J, Hill E, et al: The impact of managed behavioral healthcare on the costs of psychiatric and chemical dependency treatment. Behavioral Healthcare Tomorrow 3:18–30, 1994

Hay/Huggins Company: Psychiatric Benefits in Employer-Provided Healthcare Plans: 1992 Report. Washington, DC, National Association of Psychiatric Health Systems, 1992

National Association of Psychiatric Health Systems: 1995 Annual Survey: Final Report. Washington, DC, National Association of Psychiatric Health Systems, 1995

Parker S, Knoll JL III: Partial hospitalization: an update. Am J Psychiatry 147:156–160, 1990

Reed SK, Hennessy KD, Mitchell OS, et al: A mental health capitation program, II: cost-benefit analysis. Hospital and Community Psychiatry 45:1097–1103, 1994

Rofman ES, Curran RF: Initiating a capitated program for HMO patients. Gen Hosp Psychiatry 17:278–284, 1995

Additional Readings

Astrachan BM, Astrachan JH: Economics of practice and inpatient care. Gen Hosp Psychiatry 11:313–319, 1989

Bond GR: An economic analysis of psychosocial rehabilitation. Hospital and Community Psychiatry 35:356–360, 1984

Clark RE, Fox TS: A framework for evaluating the economic impact of case management. Hospital and Community Psychiatry 44:469–473, 1993

Dorwart RA, Hoover CW: A national study of transitional hospital services in mental health. Am J Public Health 84:1229–1234, 1994

Friedman RM: Mental health and substance abuse services for adolescents: clinical and service system issues. Administration and Policy in Mental Health 19:159–178, 1992

15 Case Management and Clinical Decision Making

Paul R. McCarthy, Ph.D.
Dorothy E. Dugger, M.D.
Arthur Lazarus, M.D.

In the era of managed care, a clinician must manage patients' care or have it managed by a third party. Clinical decision making in a managed care environment requires attention to a variety of variables not previously considered central to clinical care. These variables include the adoption of a broader systems perspective, attention to issues of accountability, and awareness of the reality of limited resources. The totality of this constellation of variables must be factored into clinical decision making.

Traditionally in private practice, the focus of treatment centered primarily on the guiding question, What can I do for my patient, given my training and expertise, that is consistent with my theoretical orientation? In general, concerns regarding the

"value" of care and the assessment and documentation of time-
liness, effectiveness, or efficiency of the treatment services rendered were absent. Instead, treatment was considered in terms
of an optimal plan designed to address all issues, often including
those problems whose etiology was primarily socioeconomic or
cultural. Beyond a consideration of the use of an inpatient versus
outpatient treatment setting, no systematic assessment of improvement was made against well-documented and operationalized ob-
servable goals. No assessment of the level of care occurred.

For treatment providers with experience in the community
mental health movement, however, managed care–era decision
making differs very little from the characteristic mode of clinical
decision making for the community mental health system. Managed care has been described as the community mental health
movement with money. Community mental health and managed
behavioral health care have a common philosophy that emphasizes the careful use of treatment resources and utilization of the
full continuum of care. Essentially, the principles of clinical decision making in the community mental health movement, including treatment at the least restrictive level of care consistent
with safety, effectiveness, and availability in the community, are
the guiding principles of managed care.

Basic to working within a managed care environment is the
need to share certain philosophies underlying managed care.
First is an orientation toward the provision of care at the least
restrictive level of care appropriate to each individual patient. A
second shared orientation focuses on the provision of care employing time-sensitive, goal-focused treatment approaches. Finally, a continuous focus on the best treatment practices targeted
to enhancing patient functioning must be a shared philosophy
of care provider and care manager.

Clinical Decision Making

Managing care in the cost-conscious environment of the present
and the future requires care providers to weigh clinical factors,

delivery system issues, and financial and resource concerns together in their clinical decision making. As outlined in Table 15–1, clinical decisions, in all cases, must incorporate the following: 1) a broad systems perspective; 2) the differentiation of medical versus social, necessary versus desirable, realistic versus ideal; 3) maintenance of a near-term, goal-directed focus, as well as awareness of the long-term needs of the patient; 4) accountability for the choice and outcome of treatment; 5) maximizing health care value (i.e., benefit of services/cost of services); and 6) consistent criteria for decisions regarding the level of care, length of stay, or the method, duration, and frequency of treatment.

Viewing systems in a broader perspective may be the most challenging transition for individual providers. The provider of care not only must think in terms of What can I do for this patient? but also must consider Where in the spectrum of mental health and/or chemical dependency services does this patient need to access appropriate care? Accordingly, the traditional practitioner must broaden his or her view of potentially therapeutic interventions to include community and public sector or other socioeconomic sources.

Table 15–1. Clinical decision-making factors for a managed care environment

---

Broad systems perspective

Differentiate:
  Medical versus social needs of the patient
  Necessary versus desirable care
  Realistic versus ideal goals in treatment planning

Time-sensitive, goal-directed treatment focus

Accountability for the choice of treatment and the outcome of care

Maximize value of care

Utilize consistent criteria for decisions regarding:
  Level of care
  Length of stay
  Duration and frequency of care

Another equally difficult challenge is differentiating between medical and social needs, necessary and desirable treatment, and realistic plans and ideal plans of patient care. A corollary to these distinctions is determining to which system each case belongs. It is important to identify clear accountability for specific services. Given the multiple systems active in providing mental health services, it is necessary to determine responsibility for certain (nonmedical) services. For example, a child with a learning disability may need intelligence testing for appropriate school programming. However, this evaluative service falls within the purview of the public educational system and is mandated by the federal government. Additionally, it is essential that responsibility is shared to ensure the coordination and systematic "handoff" of a clinical case to each appropriate agency. For example, although it may be socially desirable to keep a patient in the hospital an additional 3 days waiting for a bed to become available at a halfway house, it may not be medically necessary. In this case, alternative temporary placement should be identified. It is a primary goal of good case management to avoid disposition problems by planning proactively, beginning at the point of evaluation and treatment planning or hospital admission. In the case of a hospitalized patient with an Axis I diagnosis of bipolar disorder and an Axis II diagnosis of narcissistic personality disorder, it may be desirable to address both conditions. However, it may be necessary only to treat the Axis I disorder to return the patient to his or her premorbid level of functioning (and, in fact, may completely satisfy the needs and agenda of the patient). Although the provider may want ideally to help the patient reach his or her maximum functioning, it may not be a realistic goal. Furthermore, it is necessary for care providers and managers to evaluate carefully whether an individual case is approaching a point of diminishing returns, wherein little or no additional demonstrable improvement accrues despite ongoing treatment.

Although specific theoretical orientations are not excluded from practice within managed behavioral care, it is fundamental to the successful operation of any form of managed care paradigm that treatment is delivered with a time-sensitive, goal-focused perspective. Although treatment modalities that have been developed with specific attention to treatment duration and intensity, such as pharmacological interventions and forms of behavior therapy, are favorably received by managed care organizations, modifications of many treatment approaches to enhance the time-sensitive nature of treatment (e.g., short-term dynamic therapies) are congruent with managed care goals. Treatment must be driven by well-articulated, specific goals achievable within a focused temporal framework. For example, a vague treatment goal such as "help patient to resolve early life conflicts resulting in current difficulties" is insufficient. Rather, a more specific goal such as "reduce patient's daily hand washing by 50% over next six sessions (3 weeks) using combination of medication and behavior therapy" aids case management and provides clear markers against which treatment progress can be measured. It must be noted that although objective treatment goals are necessary, they must be employed flexibly because patients progress at different rates.

The emphasis on the issue of accountability in health care is relatively recent. Historically, care provision systems rapidly expanded, proliferating in number, size, and complexity. Although considerable advances in the science and the delivery of care resulted from this expansion, the costs of care also ballooned wildly. In response to runaway costs, a wide variety of cost-containment methodologies were developed. It is against this backdrop that managed care began. With an early, nearly exclusive focus on managing health care dollars, these organizations worked to control the expenses associated with overbuilt care provision systems. Although some progress has been made at slowing the spiraling costs of care, there is widespread concern that the quality of care may be sacrificed in the name of cost containment. A new and growing concern about health care quality has resulted in a current focus on assessment and accountability. To this end, each clinician must provide treatment with a continual awareness of several questions central to the practice of modern health care.

First, of all the alternative treatments available, what form of treatment will likely work best for the patient? With more than 150 different forms of mental health and chemical dependency treatments being used today, behavioral health care providers must be accountable for choosing a form of treatment that is appropriate for each patient's problem(s). This clinical care responsibility necessitates that health care providers work actively to keep abreast of current clinical practice and research. Second, is the patient actually benefiting from the treatment(s) he or she is receiving? This question focuses on the efficacy of treatment. Clinicians are responsible for evaluating and documenting improvement resulting from the care they deliver. Finally, is the patient receiving the most value for the health care dollars being expended? Thus, the health care provision system (e.g., provider, group) must be accountable for the selection of treatment and its delivery, as well as its outcome and cost.

Approaches to treatment that emphasize the ideal and the desirable must be compared with treatment that seeks to emphasize the value of care. The concept of health care value emphasizes not merely the costs of care or exclusively the amount of improvement yielded by treatment. Instead, the value of care is a ratio of the degree of improvement relative to the amount of health care dollars expended on treatment. Accordingly, a treatment may be highly effective, accomplishing notable improvement. Yet, if this treatment requires significantly greater health care cost, it may impart less value than a moderately effective treatment delivered in a more cost-effective manner.

Case Management

Case management and utilization review functions are changing dramatically. The importance of allocating health care resources properly has never been more apparent. Perhaps the typical clinician's exposure to care managers and utilization reviewers has been as direct agents of managed care organizations. However, managed care is progressing through yet another generation. Providers and care provision systems are now shifting from earlier fee-for-service arrangements to shared-risk or full-risk contracts for large populations of people. In light of this change, the function of case management and utilization management is moving away from managed care organizations and instead is being performed by providers of care.

Case management is an expensive health care service. Thus, it must be utilized in a manner to maximize its value to the care provision system. As a resource, case management is used for the full range of facility-based care, including acute inpatient, residential treatment, and partial hospital medical care. However, the intensity and frequency of case management may decrease with the intensity of the level of care. Utilization review is not routinely conducted on outpatient levels of care. However, utilization review may be effective for outpatient cases to enhance the value of care for patients with complex and/or chronic, recurring disorders.

Case management focuses on both the concurrent and proactive planning of care. The care manager attempts to work collegially with providers to help establish care plans that are clinically and resource sensitive. Furthermore, by design, case management seeks to ensure longer periods of quality care and prevent readmissions and relapses.

Basic Guidelines

Ideally, for the provider or provider group, the boundaries blur between clinical decision making and utilization/case management concerns, helping to shape the practice of each clinician. Care managers work to help providers better define their treatment planning goals.

Clinical decision making and case management in a managed care environment begin at the earliest point of entry into the system. History taking for each patient should be detailed, and symptoms should be described in specific, quantifiable terms. Thus, a problem that reads, "patient upset due to the loss of spouse" is better stated as, "patient experiencing depression with sleep disturbance (sleep onset problem, latency at 1–3 hours), appetite loss with corresponding weight loss (6 lb), and daily tearfulness (8–10 times/day) due to the loss of spouse to cancer 3 months ago." Many of the best provider systems accomplish this by using standardized evaluation protocols, requiring all major factors to be addressed while allowing sufficient latitude for assessing specific problems. Although many providers have improved significantly in the extent and specificity of their documentation of symptoms, it is important that psychosocial and family issues also be evaluated and addressed. A comprehensive substance abuse history should be taken for each patient. The failure to detect substance abuse has often resulted in ineffective patent care. In addition, a mental status examination should be conducted for each case, with findings documented in clear and objective terms.

To enable sound clinical decision making, the clinical formulation of each case must be clear and well reasoned. The manager of care works with providers to ensure that this formulation is well articulated and explicated in case documentation. The diagnosis for each patient must be consistent with that patient's history and mental status results. Diagnoses must directly relate to and follow from the clinical formulation of the case. The diagnosis (or diagnoses) for a patient should correspond to the criteria for that disorder as outlined in DSM-IV (American Psychiatric Association 1994a) and be clearly supported by the clinical evidence. In formulating the treatment plan, the recommended treatment modality must be appropriate for the patient. For example, although cognitively oriented treatment may be generally appropriate for depression, a particular patient may be sufficiently depressed that he or she lacks the necessary cognitive capacity to comply with that treatment approach. Clearly, a primary focus for such a case includes a psychopharmacological intervention. The treatment goals for each case should be clear and specific. These goals are best stated in behavioral terms. Instead of defining a treatment goal as "increased self-esteem," identify the specific aspect of improved function (e.g., greater participation in group meetings in the workplace) as a goal for treatment. The treatment goals and the target dates must fit within the conceptualization of a short-term treatment plan. The complete elimination of a complex disorder is not a reasonable goal because it is not time sensitive. Instead, goals focused on diminishing specific aspects of the disorder and enhancing the patient's functioning are better. The treatment interventions chosen in a patient's treatment plan must be specific to the goal as stated in the plan. Furthermore, periodic reevaluations and changes in the treatment plan should occur routinely, as well as second opinions and consultations as needed. There must be evidence of clear and frequent communication and complementary treatment with other providers, both medical and nonmedical.

Criteria

Until recently, managed care organizations and insurers had their own sets of criteria by which providers of care were expected to make level of care decisions. However, payers and employers look progressively toward capitated provider groups to develop level of care criteria or to self-administer the managed care organization's guidelines. Among most managed care organizations, criteria sets for level of care decisions have remarkably similar content. For example, for the majority of managed care criteria sets, inpatient care is judged to be medically necessary if patients represent an active immediate danger to themselves or others, are unable to care for themselves, or have failed to respond to treatment at a less intensive level. These criteria sets generally parallel clinical decision making of most providers working in vertically integrated multidisciplinary settings.

For a provider group choosing to develop their own criteria sets for admission, continued stay, and discharge from various levels of care, a synthesis of available existing criteria is well grounded and expedient. A provider group can review published criteria sets from CIGNA, Value Behavioral Health, and Green Spring Health Services (among others), extracting common criteria for inpatient, residential, partial hospital, intensive outpatient, group home, and outpatient care (most managed care organizations make their criteria available to members of their provider network). It is important to have criteria for all levels of care along the treatment continuum, regardless of whether the provider system offers that service and whether the payer considers it to be an eligible benefit. Additionally, it is critical to document all level of care decisions based on the criteria used. This decision process, and its documentation, becomes an integral part of the provider quality program and may serve as a basis for appealing noncertified treatment.

To demonstrate consistency and efficacy of treatment, standardized screening and triage forms are necessary with clear criteria, based on clinical outcomes research. Treatment plans, although individualized, must also reflect the current knowledge in clinical outcomes, and appropriate expertise needs to be available for the treatment of a wide range of disorders. This can be consistent with the use of standard practice guidelines (e.g., MCC Behavioral Care has published practice guidelines for its providers) or critical clinical pathways for the treatment of specific disorders.

Clinical Pathways

The concept of "critical paths" in the practice of medicine has received considerable attention lately. Clinical guidelines or pathways have been defined as "systematically developed statements to assist practitioner decisions about appropriate health care for specific clinical circumstances" (Grimshaw and Russell 1993, p. 1317). Although a "best practices" mandate has been opposed by many providers of care, there are some clear, well-researched and documented practices and treatments for (some) specific mental health/chemical dependency disorders. The appropriate and timely utilization of these practices improves the likelihood of a positive outcome. Several clear examples are the timely use of antidepressant medications for patients experiencing major depression, using lithium and similar mood-stabilizing drugs for bipolar patients, and employing serotonin reuptake blocking agents in conjunction with exposure and response prevention with obsessive-compulsive patients. The literature is expanding rapidly with standards of treatment in the form of clinical guidelines and practice parameters. Use of these clinical guidelines and pathways for specific disorders aids in reducing the extremes of variation in treatment practices. Although a review of the available clinical guidelines for mental health and chemical dependency disorders is beyond the scope of this chapter, the reader may find the review of several well-developed and widely recognized clinical guidelines instructive, for example, *Depression in Primary Care* (Public Health Service, Agency for Health Care Policy and Research 1993) and *Practice Guideline for the Treatment of Patients With Bipolar Disorder* (American Psychiatric Association 1994b).

Organizational Issues

The key components of vertically integrated systems of care include inpatient, residential, partial hospital, intensive outpatient, outpatient, emergency services, alternative living arrangements, and home care. Although a provider group may not deliver all services on this continuum, a detailed working knowledge of these services, as well as how to access them in the community, is important to effective functioning. In addition, the provider must be aware of community (e.g., school, church, self-help), public sector, and other legal and financial resources available to the patient population.

A provider group must be organized to address the distinctive nature of the current mental health system. As compared with medical-surgical practice, there is no single point of assessment and triage. Treatment of specific disorders is more variable, depending on the provider's professional training and theoretical orientation (e.g., biological, behavioral, cognitive, analytical).

Information management systems are key to facilitating treatment in managed care delivery systems. A care provision system needs to track numerous forms for quality assurance, level of care decisions, assessment and triage to specific providers, and clinical practice guidelines and outcomes assessment, as well as standardized intake forms, treatment plans, and case notes. It is possible to have a paper system in which all of this information is recorded and stored. However, functions such as information retrieval, measurement and tracking, and communication of this information among multiple providers and across multiple sites become costly and time consuming for a practice without a well-designed information management system. Ideally, all standardized forms and the patient clinical record should be on-line. In the future, many managed care organizations hope to provide contracted providers with on-line criteria and practice parameters for their office or group. This will enable health care providers to compare a patient's clinical data with level of care criteria. Thus, the managed care organization may be contacted by the clinician for peer review only if the proposed treatment plan is not in accord with the standard criteria. Currently, some providers with automated patient records allow the payer's utilization management personnel to review case records by modem, using a security code that restricts access to the case records of only the patients for whom they are responsible. Utilization management decisions can be entered, and only those cases not certified on the basis of the case record need be reviewed by telephone. This offers the clear advantage of saving review time and costs for both the provider and the managed care organization.

Services and Staffing

Even if the only major service being provided is outpatient treatment, it is essential for a provider group to include the capacity for emergency evaluations. Especially in the areas of detoxification and the management of mental illnesses requiring use of medications, psychiatric outpatient treatment may well be effective in stabilizing a patient, enabling treatment at a less intensive and restrictive level of care. The timely access to psychiatric evaluation and treatment can be a key distinguishing feature in providing appropriate, high-quality, cost-effective treatment with good outcomes. This issue becomes especially relevant if the provider system is capitated for the entire continuum of care for a group of patients. The cost and quality implications necessitate access to a multidisciplinary composition of providers. It is a clear and stated preference for managed care systems to contract with a multidisciplinary group offering "one-stop shopping." The solo provider or small group of homogeneous providers may become more desirable to managed care organizations through partnerships, joint ventures, or marketing alliances with complementary providers and sites for the continuum of clinical services and better geographic coverage.

Given the rapid consolidation among managed care organizations and insurers, it is likely that large physician-hospital organizations, whether organized at a local, regional, or national level, will become the preferred recipients of a large number of patients enrolled in managed care plans.

Conclusion

Managed care has progressed considerably since its advent. As it matures into what has been termed *fourth-generation managed care,* it will continue to become more clinically sensitive, and the systems delivering this care will grow more comprehensive and integrated. Within this changing environment, case management and utilization review will likely return to the purview of the provider of care. Clinicians will form large vertically integrated delivery systems, providing the full continuum of treatment services with wide geographic access to care. These integrated delivery systems, financed by full-risk capitation contracts for large populations, will demonstrate high levels of health care value, effective data management, and superior intra- and intersystem communication.

References

American Psychiatric Association: Diagnostic and Statistical Manual of Mental Disorders, 4th Edition. Washington, DC, American Psychiatric Association, 1994a

American Psychiatric Association: Practice guideline for the treatment of patients with bipolar disorder. Am J Psychiatry 151 (suppl 12):1–36, 1994b

Grimshaw JM, Russell IT: Effects of clinical guidelines on medical practice: a systematic review of rigorous evaluations. Lancet 2:1317–1322, 1993

Public Health Service, Agency for Health Care Policy and Research: Depression in Primary Care, Vols 1 and 2 (Clinical Practice Guideline No 5). Rockville, MD, U.S. Department of Health and Human Services, Public Health Service, 1993

Additional Readings

American Psychiatric Association: Practice Guideline for Major Depressive Disorder in Adults. Washington, DC, American Psychiatric Press, 1993

Bickler JB, Gartner C, Lindeman B: Managed healthcare organizational readiness guide and checklist (Special Rep). Rockville, MD, U.S. Department of Health and Human Services, Center for Substance Abuse Treatment, 1994

Gray GV, Glazer WM: Psychiatric decision making in the 90s: the coming era of decision support. Behavioral Healthcare Tomorrow 3:47–54, 1994

Lemieux-Charles L, Meslin EM, Aird C, et al: Ethical issues faced by clinician/managers in resource-allocation decisions. Hospital and Health Services Administration 38:267–285, 1993

McCarthy PR, Gelber S, Dugger DE: Outcome measurement to outcome management: the critical step. Administration and Policy in Mental Health 21:59–68, 1993

Ransohoff J: Probing the "mystery" of behavioral case management. Behavioral Health Management 14:29–30, 1994

16 Computer Decision-Support as a Clinician's Tool

H. Edmund Pigott, Ph.D.

Mr. S was a 42-year-old male referred to the mobile crisis team by a homeless shelter because of his bizarre and threatening behavior toward staff, other occupants, and himself. Mr. S was laid off 9 months ago from a factory job he had held for 23 years. His wife of 22 years left him and moved in with her parents, taking with her their two teenage children, after the family had been evicted from their home last month. Mr. S was very disheveled in appearance, reported not sleeping for several days, was moderately coherent, and complained of hearing derogatory voices in his head. Mr. S admitted threatening others because he believed that someone had stolen the watch his wife had given him for their 20th wedding anniversary. Mr. S acknowledged having intermittent thoughts of wanting to kill himself by jumping off the Oak Street bridge ever since his wife and children moved out. He then stated that he wavered in his intent to act on this plan because

245

of its effects on his family and because of his religious convictions.

The crisis team input the data into the Department of Mental Health's expert decision-support software system. Mr. S's risk severity profile placed him in the profound range on the suicidal severity subscale, moderate range on psychotic severity, and extreme range for psychosocial stressors. His overall psychiatric acuity level was in the profound range. This risk severity level required an intensity of care involving extensive daily contact, 24-hour-a-day accessibility, and an immediate psychiatric evaluation to review the treatment plan. Care options for this intensity of care level included inpatient hospitalization, a respite/holding bed, intensive in-home services, and an on-site holding bed.

The on-call psychiatrist evaluated the patient and started him on trazodone for sleep. She concurred with the team's plan to implement a structured on-site holding bed at the shelter and agreed to reassess the patient the next morning. The team had also contacted the patient's wife, who agreed to meet with them the next day. The team chose this care option because of the acute onset of the patient's condition and their desire to avert hospitalization due to its potential iatrogenic consequences for the patient.

Real incidents—similar to those presented in this vignette—occur thousands of times each day and make behavioral health a $75-billion-per-year industry in this country. The clinical decisions of more than 100,000 behavioral health professionals directly affect the quality of outcomes patients receive and the cost to receive it.

Behavioral health providers face a daunting social obligation: as the growth in the continuum of care accelerates, so does the challenge to make appropriate use of it. It is no longer a simple decision between inpatient versus outpatient care for our patients. The number of treatment options providers must choose from is steadily increasing, equally driven by clinical advances and health care economics. Many of the patients in the case vignettes in this book—which the authors selected to illustrate individuals uniquely suited for their service—could be shuffled like cards and dealt to a different service with perhaps equally impressive outcomes. Imagine the overlap in patients if we considered the full range of cases each program serves.

Authoritative rationales are generated either on an a priori or a post hoc basis for almost any clinical decision. This fact causes wide variance in clinical practice across professions, across providers within a specific profession, and even within individual providers (e.g., on Monday morning, the way you handle a suicidal patient who has one insurance plan probably differs from the way you handle an identical patient with different insurance late on Friday afternoon when you are preparing to leave for the weekend).

This variance in clinical practice results in widely varying types and costs of care, as well as clinical outcomes, for patients with similar conditions. Such wide variance is due to the historical failure by the behavioral health professions to systematically link patient assessment data, and their analysis, to actual clinical decision making. This discontinuity has severely stymied progress in behavioral health as compared with other medical specialties that strive to make such linkages quite explicit.

The virtually unrestrained, and at times celebrated, variance in behavioral health practice is the principal cause of our peculiar paradox. This paradox is the fact that despite 40 years of solid biopsychosocial research documenting the direct and indirect value of defined behavioral health services, the behavioral health field is still the orphaned child pleading to end payer's discrimination against our patients and ourselves while our health care siblings look on, bemused by our struggle.

To address this issue and decrease such variance, expert software systems have been developed by managed care companies to ensure consistency in their case managers' level of care authorizations. In this chapter, I describe a provider-driven approach to developing a decision-support software tool to enhance the quality and consistency of providers' clinical decision making. It is my contention that systematically linking essential patient data to providers' actual clinical decision making—and integrating these data into outcomes analysis—will not only accelerate advances in our field but strengthen behavioral health's argument for parity in health care benefits.

Expert System Developers' Clinical Biases and Objectives

In developing any expert system, it is critical that the "experts" be explicit about their own clinical biases and objectives for the system. The developers of PATHware, an expert system I helped develop, had seven explicit biases and objectives (along with some unconscious/unstated ones, I am sure). These were 1) the hazards of overtreatment are potentially as deleterious to the long-term functioning of patients as the hazards of undertreatment; 2) patient risk factors are the de facto driver of level and intensity of care decision making; 3) most behavioral health providers' unspoken (and, for some, unconscious) belief is that more care is better care; 4) providers need to be educated, equipped, and empowered to be the ultimate decision maker for their patients because they have the maximum impact on the quality and cost of care; 5) nonpsychiatric providers are increasingly performing the initial assessments of patients, even those in acute distress, yet there is no consistent means of triaging appropriate cases to psychiatrists; 6) to maximize an expert system's effectiveness and end-user acceptability, it must be easy to use, save providers' time, increase providers' confidence in their clinical decisions, and be easily modifiable, thereby permitting direct involvement by providers in shaping expert system application; and 7) historically, behavioral health providers have failed to systematically link critical patient data to differential clinical decision making, and this fact has undermined our quest for parity.

First, we believe the hazards of overtreatment are as deleterious to the long-term functioning of patients as the hazards of undertreatment. The consequences of undertreatment are well known and include the dramatic (e.g., suicide) and the more subtle (e.g., unnecessary intrapsychic and familial suffering, decreased productivity, increased medical utilization).

The potential adverse consequences of overtreatment are less well known. For instance, there is no available research indicating that inpatient hospitalization decreases patients' suicide risk beyond the length of their hospitalization. The available data indicate that patients have a high suicide rate during the first month following hospital discharge (Black et al. 1985). In fact, hospital discharge was found to be the best predictor of successful suicide. It is important to note that this study was done before the incursion of managed care into clinical decision making, when the length of stays were generally as long as providers deemed necessary.

An exhaustive review (Pigott and Trott 1993) of six controlled studies using random assignment procedures to compare inpatient hospitalization with intensive outpatient programs, including an in-home component, found the following:

- Intensive outpatient program services averted hospitalization for approximately 75% of patients.
- Patients receiving intensive outpatient program services had a 50% lower psychiatric rehospitalization rate compared with hospitalized patients.
- Patients receiving intensive outpatient program services reported greater life satisfaction and fewer psychiatric symptoms and were superior in work adjustment and ability to manage future crises.
- Of 807 patients participating in the six random assignment studies, three of 404 hospitalized patients committed suicide during the follow-up periods. There were no reports of suicide among the 403 patients receiving intensive outpatient program services.

The available data strongly suggest that psychiatric hospitalization is not a benign experience for many patients. Although hospitalization is necessary to ensure safety for some patients, for others, it appears to increase suicide risk as well as the likelihood of future psychiatric relapse/rehospitalization and diminished psychosocial functioning.

Clinical decision making is risky business. There are real risks associated with both under- and overtreatment regardless of the intensity of care decision (e.g., inpatient versus partial or partial versus intensive outpatient). Unfortunately, providers cannot look to the accepted truisms of the behavioral health field to guide their decision making because some are often quite wrong.

Second, we believe that in the current health care reimbursement environment, patient risk factors are the de facto driver in intensity of care decision making. These risk factors include the patients' potential 1) to harm themselves or others physically; 2) to engage in behaviors significantly harmful to themselves, others, and/or their relationships with others; and 3) to decompensate such that they cannot care for themselves. Most providers are inadequately trained in performing such thorough risk assessments and then effectively intervening on the identified risk factors. In general, most psychiatric evaluations and psychological testing reports are long on patient description and analysis, which is then at best weakly linked to generic treatment recommendations.

Much of the data behavioral health providers are trained to gather—although interesting and at times therapeutic—are actually "noise" in regard to clinical decision making. To allocate behavioral health resources effectively, expert systems need to be designed and implemented for systematically assessing critical patient variables linked to differential clinical decision making.

Third, we believe most behavioral health providers' unspoken belief is that more care is better care, particularly when they are the provider. Such providers tend to overtreat patients and promote dependency, thereby undermining patients' long-term functioning.

Fourth, we believe providers need to be educated, equipped, and empowered to be the ultimate decision maker for their patients. Only then can they integrate objective risk assessment data, and the resulting treatment recommendations, with their patients' unique personalities and life situations. By empowering providers to tailor treatment recommendations—within defined limits—to match their patients' unique needs best, they are able to impact the quality and cost of care maximally.

Fifth, we believe nonpsychiatric providers are increasingly performing the initial assessments of patients and then referring to psychiatrists when the nonpsychiatrist deems it appropriate. The quality of such providers' clinical judgment varies greatly, thereby raising significant risk management and quality of care issues. An expert system should identify for non-M.D. providers those cases that require an immediate psychiatric evaluation versus those that can be scheduled on a routine basis.

Sixth, we believe to maximize an expert system's effectiveness and end-user acceptability, it must be easy to use, save providers' time, increase providers' confidence in their clinical decisions, and be easily modifiable, thereby permitting direct involvement by providers in shaping the expert system application.

Finally, we believe that, historically, behavioral health providers have failed to systematically link critical patient data to differential clinical decision making. This failure has severely stymied progress in behavioral health care, in contrast to other medical specialties, and contributes to the undervaluing of our services within society.

One Model for Building Expert Decision-Support Software Applications

To address the historical failure of behavioral health providers to systematically link critical patient data to differential clinical decision making, we developed an expert system software configuration tool (PATHcfg) by which "domain experts" can directly build applications without requiring programming expertise.

PATHcfg enables such domain experts or "protocol development teams" to build software applications that model their decision-making logic for distribution to providers. The actual expert system software application distributed to providers (or end users) is called PATHware.

The first step in developing the initial PATHware application was defining its intended scope. We decided to limit the focus of the system initially to acute psychiatric clinical presentations. This patient population accounts for the 8% of all psychiatric patients who consume 70% of behavioral health dollars. Following implementation with this patient population, we hope to extend the methodology to develop applications for other patient groups and/or behavioral health "disease states."

The second step was identifying the essential risk assessment data necessary for making clinical decisions for patients who present significant risk management issues. Much patient data are wholly unique to the patient and therefore are of limited value in terms of making intensity of care decisions for at-risk patients. Such data, however, are oftentimes critical for providers in 1) forming a therapeutic alliance, 2) informing them how to present treatment recommendations, and 3) maximizing treatment compliance. The effective use of such clinical noise will always be an essential part of behavioral health providers' "art."

Assessing, and successfully intervening on, risk factors is the critical component to the science of delivering acute behavioral health services. As previously stated, patients' identified risk factors drive most providers' intensity of care decisions. A properly designed expert system can ensure consistency in the thorough assessment of such factors.

"Risk level," as used here, refers to patients' risk 1) to harm themselves or others physically; 2) to engage in behaviors significantly harmful to themselves, others, and/or their relationships with others; and 3) to decompensate such that they cannot care for themselves.

For adult patients, the crucial risk factors to assess include 1) suicidal severity, 2) homicidal severity, 3) psychotic severity,

4) grave disability, 5) substance abuse severity, 6) psychosocial stressors, and 7) general psychiatric factors.

Just as there are factors that increase a patient's risk level, there are other factors that mitigate a patient's risk level. Such factors include the patient's 1) rapport with the therapist, 2) commitment to treatment, 3) willingness to sign a "no-harm" contract and the provider's assessment of the patient's ability to adhere to it, and 4) psychosocial resources available to assist in the treatment plan.

Once the assessment factors, which are directly related to clinical decision making, are established, multiple questions are developed to assess each factor. Providing behaviorally specific response options for each question increases the likelihood of establishing adequate interrater reliability of the assessment procedure (for an example, see Figure 16–1).

Before implementation, it is essential to conduct interrater reliability studies by having multiple providers use the assessment tool to rate various patients. To measure interrater reliability, providers' ratings of the same patients are correlated item by item, and only those items that demonstrate a high correlation between raters are kept. This is the only means to establish the soundness of the assessment tool. The potential value of using

---

0:   None reported

1:   Passive, infrequent ideation

2:   Active ideation, past week

3:   Current active ideation, but with periods of relief

4:   Current and persistent ideation

Figure 16–1.   Present suicidal ideation.

---

an expert system to guide clinical decision making presupposes first that different providers rate patients in a highly similar manner using the proposed assessment tool. Establishing the assessment tool's interrater reliability is a necessary prerequisite to establishing the validity of the treatment recommendations generated by the expert system.

After identifying the questions necessary to address each factor sufficiently, and writing specific behavioral responses for questions that have high interrater reliability, expert system developers must assign differential weights to each potential response. Clinically, all information is not equal. Certain information is more important from a risk management perspective than other information. Just as active suicide intent is (or should be) weighted more heavily in providers' clinical decision making than infrequent suicidal ideation, such differential weighting must be captured in an expert system.

To establish such weightings, one strategy is to have providers independently sort into six to eight different severity categories the response options associated with each question. After all providers have completed this task, the developers can then determine each response option's correspondence rate among providers, as well as the average weighting providers assigned to each response option. Response options with a high correspondence rate indicate a high level of agreement among providers in their assigning relative importance to the response option.

Only those questions with high interrater reliability, and those for which providers assign a high level of importance to each response option, should be included in the expert system.

Figure 16–2 graphically presents a model for linking expert system decision-support to providers with ongoing outcomes analysis. The model utilizes essential intake data to identify clinical pathways that will optimally treat patients in a cost-efficient manner. The model then links the prospective focus of the selected clinical pathway with the retrospective rigor of outcomes analysis to foster the ongoing refinement of treatment recommendations.

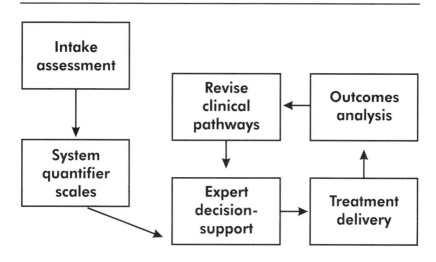

Figure 16–2.   PATHware: linking outcomes analysis to clinical pathways.

Intake Assessment

The resulting PATHware application uses a computer-assisted intake assessment to "quiz" providers with behaviorally specific items to gather data critical for clinical decision making. This assessment "branches" the administration of items based on prior responses to increase efficiency.

An expert system should provide on-line training support through a help screen format to give providers real-time assistance when they are uncertain about how to respond to a specific item. The systematic administration of items for providers to respond to, combined with follow-up items as necessary, can positively shape providers' patient assessment skills.

Finally, during the intake process, patients' level of functioning and other outcome measures should be collected as part of an ongoing outcomes analysis effort.

System Quantifier Scales

Once the intake assessment information is entered, the expert system computes patients' risk severity profiles with separate

subscale scores for each identified risk factor. The various subscale scores can then be differentially weighted to compute an
overall psychiatric acuity level (Figure 16–3). The expert system
also computes patients' risk mitigation profiles and overall risk
mitigation levels (Figure 16–4).

Finally, the system can summarize those items for each subscale that most contribute to its rating—by either increasing or
decreasing risk. This summary is crucial for providers in high-
lighting those specific item responses that heighten and/or reduce risk for patients. The summary, combined with a graphical
presentation of the subscale scores, gives providers a hard copy
of their clinical assessment and facilitates their tailoring treatment recommendations to best address the risk management
issues their patients present.

Expert System Decision-Support

The expert system then computes the overall risk severity scale
score by combining a patient's psychiatric acuity level with his
or her risk mitigation level (Figure 16–5). A patient's overall risk
severity score is then directly related to the intensity of care necessary to treat the patient while appropriately managing his or
her level of risk.

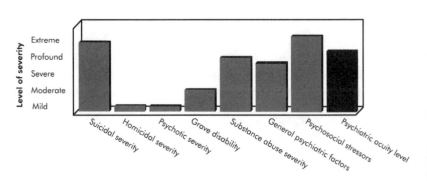

Figure 16–3. PATHware: patient risk severity profile.

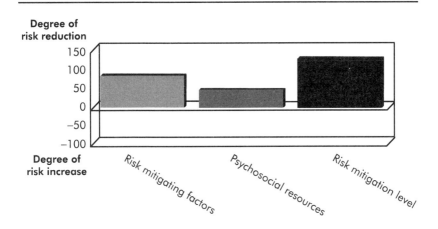

Figure 16–4.   PATHware: patient risk mitigation profile.

In Figure 16–5, the recommended intensity of care level is then matched to a range of care options available that are appropriate to manage patients' risk severity level. Providers then select from the range of care options based on unique knowledge of their patients and the patients' life situations. Naturally, the provider is able to select, based on his or her professional judgment, a care option that is not listed.

Next, the system recommends specific treatment goals and interventions based on the patient's risk severity profile and/or responses to specific assessment items. These suggested treatment goals and interventions are independent from the identified intensity of care and the selected care option. The combination of a specified intensity of care and selected care option, with specific treatment goals and interventions, constitutes the expert system's critical clinical pathway for patients.

Developing such critical clinical pathways for a behavioral health delivery system involves

● Establishing an interdisciplinary "protocol development team"

Risk severity scale	Intensity of care	Care options	Recommended goals and interventions
Extreme	24-hour professional care	• Inpatient stabilization on locked unit	Patient-specific treatment goals and interventions. These recommendations are based on the patient's risk severity profile and responses to specific items.
Profound	Extended care 5–7 days/week 24-hour immediate accessibility	• Inpatient • Respite bed • Intensive • In-home in-home holding bed	
Severe	Extended care 3–5 times/week	• In-home crisis intervention • Day treatment • Structured outpatient services • Residential treatment center (chronic)	
Moderate	2–3 times/week	• Intensive outpatient • Psychiatric home visits • Evening program	
Mild	Weekly/biweekly	• Problem-focused outpatient • Psychoeducational support groups • Support services	
Not significant	Wellness/prevention	• Problem-focused outpatient • Psychoeducational support groups • Support services	

100 ◄──────────────────────────────── 0

Figure 16–5.   PATHware: patient risk severity scale.

- Identifying the critical patient variables that the team believes (based on clinical experience, review of the research literature, and when necessary, consultation with outside experts) should drive the organization's differential decision-making process and including these variables in the initial computer-assisted intake assessment
- Developing a consensus among team members regarding specific interventions for patients with various patient profiles
- Incorporating intended end users in the development process by seeking their feedback on the emerging critical pathways under development
- Running trial cases through the emerging expert system (such cases can be assessed either by the software or a hard copy) for testing and determining necessary modifications to ensure clinical integrity and end-user acceptability

The development of such critical clinical pathways forces the organization's protocol development team to establish explicit links between presenting patient variables and differential clinical decisions. For example, with depressed patients, the team must address the following questions for the organization: Who is appropriate for cognitive-behavior therapy, interpersonal therapy, dynamic therapy, or distress tolerance training versus a trial on medication alone or in combination with one of the therapies? Who is appropriate for such treatment to be offered via individual, group, or marital/family therapy, or some combination thereof? Who is appropriate for an initial trial on a five-cent tricyclic versus a two-dollar selective serotonin reuptake inhibitor? Which patients are appropriate for the initial medication evaluation to be performed by their primary care physician versus those requiring a psychiatric evaluation (taking into account that currently 75% of all antidepressants are prescribed by primary care physicians with no rational patient routing mechanism in place)? Which depressed suicidal patients can be safely managed via a no-harm contract, telephone monitoring, and/or multiple weekly contacts versus those requiring admission on a locked inpatient unit? Which substance-abusing depressed patients should first have a 4- to 6-week period of sobriety to assess if this resolves their depression versus those who would likely benefit by initiating antidepressant therapy at the beginning of treatment? Which depressed patients likely require long-term antidepressant therapy versus just a 4- to 6-month medication trial? What differential medication compliance strategies are necessary for those patients on maintenance therapy versus a more limited medication trial?

Identifying, and defining in measurable terms, the patient variables that drive such differential decision making is critical in the development of an organization's clinical pathways. This is not to imply, however, that such pathways are to be rigidly applied. There will always be clinical situations that require the provider to select (or deselect) other treatment components. The purpose of the pathway is to make such clinical "deviations" conscious and, if they are more efficient and/or lead to superior effects, repeatable.

In the final analysis, the purpose of expert system clinical pathways is to enhance consistency in clinical decision making, thereby enabling the informed improvement of said pathways.

Treatment Delivery

The provider then takes the intake summary and suggested treatment interventions and customizes the treatment plan based on unique knowledge of the patient. The expert system records in a relational database the system-recommended, provider-planned, and actually delivered components of care. These data can then be used later for outcomes analysis.

Outcomes Analysis

At regularly scheduled intervals, the outcomes assessment measures are readministered. These measures, combined with the service delivery data, permit the evaluation of the expert system's validity. Essential data to use in assessing the expert system's validity include 1) the number of times patients have to be "bumped up" to a higher intensity of care during the first week of treatment, thereby indicating the expert system has not accurately identified the appropriate level of care; 2) the readmission/relapse rates into more intensive levels of care for patients assessed by the expert system compared with industry norms; 3) the providers' rate of concurrence/nonconcurrence with the expert system's recommended intensity of care; and 4) the quality of clinical outcomes for patients.

Over time, by conducting statistical analyses of the expert system's relational database, researchers can predict the course, cost, and resulting outcomes for patients with different risk severity profiles. Such a database then permits severity-adjusted profiling by providers and programs based on the outcomes their services produce.

Revise Clinical Pathways

An analysis of the database also can identify those patient risk profiles and their resulting clinical pathways that produce less than optimal outcomes. With such knowledge, system developers can seek outside consultation for targeted pathway revisions. The relational database can also be used to identify critical variances in provider practice patterns that are correlated with enhanced patient outcomes, thereby flagging helpful revisions to recommended clinical pathways.

Summary

The field of behavioral health care has developed in a way that is fundamentally at odds with other health care specialties. Behavioral health treatment, because of its necessary emphasis on patient confidentiality, takes place behind closed doors and is essentially a private affair between the therapist and his or patient.

Before the advent of managed care, clinical decisions were made by the patient's therapist, and to the extent that the patient concurred (and had insurance to pay for it), the treatment plan was implemented. Because a provider's clinical decisions were essentially unscrutinized, the only incentives to incorporate clinical research findings into his or her practice were intrinsic—and any hope for widespread quality assurance was a myth.

In contrast, other health care fields developed in a more "public" manner, forcing such practitioners to stay reasonably current in their respective fields. Imagine the professional life expectancy of surgeons who do not stay up-to-date with the latest surgery techniques in their area of specialization. The public nature of other health care fields reinforces conformity to established professional standards and ensures more rapid dissemination of clinical research findings. This has resulted in society's conferring great value to these practitioners and their services, as best evidenced by health insurance benefits.

The private nature of behavioral health treatment, on the other hand, has resulted in numerous "schools of psychotherapy," wide variance in clinical practice for patients with similar conditions, virtual disregard of clinical research findings by many practitioners, and a society conflicted about the value of our services.

Managed care companies were the first to bring some external scrutiny to the practice of behavioral health. Although this has enraged many providers and their patients—some rightfully so—it also has triggered a necessary process of making more "public" the practice of behavioral health.

Expert decision-support software systems open the clinical decision-making process to external scrutiny. They provide the opportunity to develop behavioral health delivery systems in which providers are equipped and empowered to act decisively in a publicly responsible manner. Key benefits include

● Enhancing the consistency of clinical decision making among providers who have widely varying professional backgrounds and levels of expertise

- Establishing clear links between assessment data and actual treatment interventions
- Making more "public" (i.e., accountable) behavioral health care practice while preserving patient confidentiality
- Providing a mechanism to ensure the rapid dissemination and implementation of new clinical research findings
- Linking the prospective focus of clinical pathways with the retrospective rigor of outcomes analysis to accelerate advances in behavioral health
- Performing severity-adjusted profiling by providers and programs based on the outcomes their services produce

Expert systems have the potential to help rectify the historical failure by the behavioral health professions to systematically link patient assessment data, and their analysis, to actual clinical decision making. Such systems will help make behavioral health practice more accountable, thereby strengthening the argument for psychiatric patients to gain parity in health care benefits.

References

Black DW, Warrack G, Winokur G: The Iowa record-linkage study: suicides and accidental deaths among psychiatric patients. Arch Gen Psychiatry 42:71–75, 1985

Pigott HE, Trott L: Curbing behavioral health costs while enhancing the quality of patient care: the implementation of a crisis intervention, triage and treatment service in the private sector. Am J Med Qual 8:138–144, 1993

17 Outcomes Management

John Bartlett, M.D., M.P.H.

In the spring of 1992, my former organization, MCC Behavioral Care, set out on a journey—a journey to create what I call an accountable, improvable approach to the delivery of behavioral care. Such an approach is characterized by clinical decision making that is based on the reasoned analysis of sound data and that, therefore, is firmly grounded in psychiatry's roots as a scientific discipline (Bartlett 1994a). More importantly, the data considered in making decisions about what constitutes appropriate care are not limited to just measures of the amount and cost of services provided but increasingly on considerations of the impact of that care on the people and systems involved. To a large extent, therefore, this journey toward accountability and improvability is designed to better define and demonstrate more clearly the value of behavioral care to a wide variety of stakeholders.

The value of behavioral care is this central question that has contributed to the phenomenal growth over the last decade of managed behavioral care programs such as the ones provided by MCC. Managed behavioral care has prospered precisely because it has been able to capitalize on the concerns about value that many payers have had under traditional indemnity programs. Recognizing that value is the relationship between the cost of a good or a service and its quality, managed care to date has leveraged the existence of alternative treatment settings and approaches along the continuum of care to decrease the cost of behavioral care and therefore impact its value positively. This willingness on the part of managed care programs to utilize and fund alternatives to traditional inpatient care and long-term psychotherapy may nowadays seem fairly routine, but many clinicians remember well how even a few years ago requests for such interventions were routinely denied on the grounds that they were not "covered" under traditional indemnity programs. In fact, such experiences were often a source of frustration for clinicians who understood that the care of many patients could actually be improved by carefully transitioning them to more independent levels of functioning (Mosher 1983). The increased availability of alternatives such as partial hospitalization and structured outpatient substance abuse programs is largely due to the increased willingness of managed care to pay for their appropriate use.

This emphasis on the financial aspects of managed care has over time led to an increasing awareness of and desire to refocus the discussion on quality. In the light of the significant savings achieved, the question more and more has become "At what cost to quality?" The marketplace's concern for quality has in turn led to an increasing emphasis on the clinical and functional results achieved under managed care. But why, one may ask, does quality equate so readily to outcomes? Outcomes is, after all, only one of the three key parameters of quality in health care (Donabedian 1980). Why is the current emphasis on quality in the behavioral health care marketplace focused almost exclusively on outcomes measurement and management rather than on the evaluation of the structures or processes of care?

The answer, I believe, lies in the wide variation in treatment approach and even philosophy that is evident among mental health and substance abuse clinicians. This wide range of approaches makes difficult, if not impossible, the development of meaningful and measurable standards of structure and process in behavioral health care. After all, what I as a managed care psychiatrist believe is good care for any given patient is most often at odds with what a practicing psychoanalyst believes. Therefore, to the extent that we want to measure and, more importantly, manage quality in demonstrable ways in our field, structural and process definitions prove inadequate. In the face of such wide variation in approach, we must in effect "cut to the chase" and measure the results of our efforts if we want to explore the nonfinancial side of the value equation. Such exploration is exactly what we as clinicians need to achieve; the alternative is to have the value of what we do measured only in financial terms and to run the risk of having the treatment of mental health and substance problems turned into a commodity, one for which purchase choices are made based on considerations of price alone.

It is important to point out, however, that the kind of quality I am talking about is not the subjective, often ill-defined concept of quality known only to a small group of insiders that has traditionally held sway in health care. Rather, it is the more objective, measurable, and ultimately improvable type of quality recognized in business and promoted under such rubrics as continuous quality improvement and total quality management (Berwick et al. 1990). Under this approach to quality, the process is one of defining objective standards and then managing the variation around them. The goal is not mindless uniformity; it is instead the reduction of waste, complexity, and rework and the continual improvement of the quality of the output of any given process through ongoing collection and analysis of its results.

In an earlier volume, I described one phase of MCC's journey toward accountability and improvability: the development and implementation of objective, documented practice guidelines (Bartlett 1994b). I characterized that effort as an attempt to reduce the variability in clinical practice by providing a set of tools to appropriately inform the therapeutic component of clinical judgment, that which addresses the question, What is the best treatment for his or her condition? Practice guidelines, when developed and implemented correctly, should represent the consensus of clinical experts using both the available empirical research and their experience. Simply put, documented clinical standards can potentially prove useful in reducing the variability evident today in clinical practice and in doing so can actually enhance quality.

Under the new quality program, therefore, the generation and documentation of clinical standards is a start to the process of defining and enhancing quality, but only a start. Having objective, documented clinical guidelines by no means relieves us of the ongoing responsibility of continually asking if they are correct. As I have already pointed out, such guidelines represent at best the current state of knowledge. As scientists and clinicians, we must be willing to ask if the guidelines in fact reflect some empirically based truth or if they are merely a distillation of current opinion. A good example from behavioral care would be the change in any hypothetical set of clinical guidelines addressing appropriate treatment for obsessive-compulsive disorder before and after the appearance of clomipramine. Documented clinical standards, such as practice guidelines, are only a first step in the journey toward accountability and improvability. They can to a greater or lesser extent address the variability in the structures and processes of care, but to be sure that they are correct, they must be combined with an effort to examine the results of their application, the outcomes, to serve as a true foundation for quality in behavioral structure.

This kind of outcomes management initiative, then—one designed to measure and evaluate the structures and processes of care by measuring their results—has been the focus of MCC's journey toward accountability and improvement. The goal of the journey has always been not just to *prove* that we had already done our work, but more importantly, to lay the foundation to *improve* what we could do in the future. The major challenge at the start lay in overcoming the fact that MCC was data rich in the financial area but, like most if not all health care organizations, was largely bankrupt in the clinical realm. We did have a large and sophisticated financial information management system that tracked and aggregated literally hundreds of thousands of individual revenue and expense transactions every year. These transaction-level data are routinely collected and aggregated into a variety of financial databases (e.g., the authorization and, separately, the claims database). These databases in turn are used to build a variety of decision-support tools, such as monthly operating reports, pricing and underwriting analyses, and patient-specific program information.

Before we started our journey, however, the clinical activities were managed largely on a case-by-case basis. Unlike financial data, the collection and aggregation of which was automated and on-line, clinical data were handwritten in narrative, nonstructured formats, with little to no aggregation of specific case-level data into standardized databases. Attempts to analyze clinical quality involved not the on-line analysis of large bodies of information but rather the laborious and often subjective review of a sample of charts to identify problems retrospectively. The analogous situation would be to attempt to run the financial affairs of a multimillion-dollar business by occasionally auditing a bill or two or by reviewing and recording every thousandth claim.

What has this journey toward accountability and quality improvement been like to date? First and foremost it has been a journey of learning, learning not just a new set of technical skills required to measure and manage clinical quality and outcomes but also the organizational processes and culture required to support such an effort. At the heart of the effort has been our attempt to build better data and information sources about clinical quality in general and outcomes in particular and, more importantly, to promote their routine use and application within the organization to drive sounder, more empirically based clinical decision making. To date, we have identified four distinct stages in the development of such an accountable, improvable approach to delivering clinical services, each of which presents a unique set of challenges and opportunities.

The first of these four stages I call the methodological stage, where the scientific and technical challenges of generating sound data about clinical outcomes must be successfully addressed. This stage is crucial because to be useful for identifying opportunities for improvement and change the information produced must be methodologically sound and believable. In short, it must be *actionable.* In measuring health care outcomes, the generation of sound data is subject to a number of threats that are well known to health services researchers. These threats include identifying valid and reliable measures to follow, generating data at both baseline and follow-up so that a measure of change can be generated, minimizing sampling bias at both baseline and follow-up, and defining and collecting meaningful data about patient-specific areas that may themselves contribute to treatment results (so-called case-mix data).

When I arrived at MCC in 1988, the organization was already struggling with the challenges of this stage. MCC had been started by clinicians in 1974 and had always run a variety of internal clinical programs, most notably some of the earliest and arguably the finest structured outpatient substance abuse treatment programs in the country. As a condition of licensure for our Minnesota-based treatment programs, MCC was routinely required by the state to report on a variety of "outcomes" areas. This effort had been conducted for a number of years with little to no methodological rigor, largely centering around attempts to contact patients who had completed the program within the previous 3 months. This effort to contact patients routinely generated among those who could be located a 50%–60% response rate to a set of nonstandardized questions. There was no baseline assessment against which to measure change, no sampling strategy, no reliability/validity assessment of the instrument, and no case-mix or severity adjustment to aid in the analysis of the data that were produced. Despite these severe methodological limitations, what was being accomplished satisfied all the requirements of the state. The difficulty lay in the fact that it was purely a bureaucratic activity being conducted for compliance reasons only; it had no management or program impact and, in fact, was incapable of driving either change or improvement. Year after year data were collected, formatted for submission to the state, and promptly forgotten.

Shortly after I arrived as corporate medical director, the organization identified the need to measure and track the cost-effectiveness of our clinical programs, including our substance abuse programs, for internal budgeting and planning reasons. Knowing that our then-current approaches to measuring treatment results were methodologically unsound, we began searching for opportunities to improve them. Fortunately, the opportunity soon arose to work with one of the country's leading behavioral health services researchers, Dr. Rick Smith, and his group from the University of Arkansas. We saw this collaboration as a chance to better understand the opportunities and challenges of conducting state-of-the-art outcomes evaluation in the "real world" of clinical practice. The specific opportunity was to help Dr. Smith and his group with the reliability and validity testing of a newly developed instrument to assess outcomes in the treatment of panic disorder.

Built into the process was the additional opportunity to conduct a traditional outcomes research study, in this case of longitudinal design, involving patients presenting for the treatment of panic disorder in a managed care setting. The study was designed to build on a body of work that had already demonstrated a decrease in the quality of life in individuals with the targeted condition. The working hypothesis of the research team was that because panic disorder has clearly defined treatments that have been shown in randomized clinical trials to be efficacious, treatment of the disorder in the clinical practice setting would be associated with demonstrable increases in quality of life. In addition, the group postulated that treatment delivered in accordance with a set of "best practices" would increase quality of life and health status more than other forms of treatment.

By the end of the study period, which lasted more than 24 months from the initial design phase through data collection to final analysis, we had learned a great deal. We learned, for example, that the overwhelming majority of patients got better, both in terms of their quality of life and their symptoms. In addition, we learned that in the managed care settings involved, most patients received care consistent with the best practices identified in the literature. In addition, although the longitudinal, nonrandomized study design did not allow us to "prove" that it was the treatment (rather than, for example, the passage of time alone) that was responsible for the improvements, the fact that the patients who did have care consistent with identified best practices demonstrated greater improvement than those who did not supported the notion that treatment did contribute to outcome for these individuals.

More importantly for MCC, we learned that doing methodologically sound outcomes studies in the clinical practice environment was laborious, inefficient, and extremely intrusive. It took many months to identify appropriate patients and collect sound data. The whole project extended almost 3 years from design to completion of the final analysis. Publication of an appropriate report in a refereed journal added an additional year and a half. For research purposes, these time frames may well be acceptable; for business and clinical decision making, they are too long by an order of magnitude. From this experience, then, we learned that although we needed to evaluate outcomes in a rigorous and methodologically sound manner, we were not in the business of researching outcomes but rather in the business of managing them as a core part of our business of managing care.

Understanding this distinction between outcomes research and outcomes management is the key to the next stage of the journey toward accountability and improvability, which I call the organizational stage. The distinction lies in recognizing the different units or building blocks on which the two rely. Research is based on an individual study; the research and the study are each freestanding and even isolated by design, to better control all parameters of the study to drive a "purer" understanding of cause and effect. Although isolation and control are essential from the scientific point of view, they directly contradict the very purpose of an outcomes management system, which is to identify opportunities to improve care. Outcomes management systems, therefore, cannot be built on individual studies because a study, no matter how methodologically sound it is, can address only a single question (or, more properly, negate a single null hypothesis). Although a study can prove that what has already happened worked, it cannot be used to improve things demonstrably. Once its results are used to drive any changes, they are essentially negated because the conditions that produced them no longer exist.

Outcomes management systems, therefore, not only must produce actionable data, but they also must do so on an outgoing, continuous basis to identify opportunities for improvement and to evaluate results of any changes made in the name of improvement. Just as the financial management systems of organizations track and aggregate transaction-level information over time, so must clinical information management systems. To accomplish this, however, the collection of sound data about outcome domains of interest must become part of the routine of the organization. It cannot be seen as an add-on but rather as a core process within the overall activities of the organization.

What then are the major challenges of this organizational stage of the journey toward accountability and improvement? They in general involve identifying the business and cultural roadblocks to building the collection of methodologically sound outcomes data into the routine processes of the organization. The greatest challenge is to avoid layering the outcomes management effort onto the already complicated and often burdensome tasks that managed care organizations require clinicians and patients to perform. The outcomes management system must be designed in a way that not only increases the value of the information gathered, but also decreases (ideally) the work required to produce it. At MCC, we have tried hard to benefit from the lessons we learned from the "research" effort I have described. Working with a group of health services researchers and industrial engineers from the University of Minnesota, we have focused our efforts on not just the methodological rigor of our data, but more importantly on engineering the collection of that data into the routine work of our organization (Pothoff et al. 1994).

For example, in structuring the collection of baseline data about substance abuse patients and their treatments for our clinical information management system, we have made a number of choices that were driven as much by the realities of the clinical work we are trying to accomplish as by the science of outcomes evaluation. These choices often involve striking an appropriate compromise between the structure and rigor required by working with patients. It is for this reason that we chose, for example, to use neither existing structured research questionnaires (the preferred scientific approach) nor retrospective chart reviews (the preferred quality assurance approach) to collect our baseline data. Formal questionnaires, although providing the greatest amount of structure, are far too rigid for routine clinical practice. Retrospective chart reviews, although they do not alter traditional clinical work flows (and therefore have been the traditional data collection approach in clinical quality), require laborious and often incomplete structuring of that data for the purposes of outcomes assessment. At MCC, we have chosen instead an approach somewhere between the two on the continuum of structure and flexibility. We have developed a standardized clinical database and history form that provides for recording both the structured, aggregatable data on a wide variety of clinical and functional areas of interest for outcomes management and the narrative entries that are so essential to the clinician's understanding of his or her patient. This structured data collection tool allows the flexibility our clinicians need to work with patients in the clinical setting while also providing the structure required to measure change and aggregate the data from literally thousands of patients into an outcomes database.

The approach works as follows: At MCC, we believe that an adequate and appropriate baseline assessment of an employed patient who is chemically dependent should include an evaluation of the impact of the patient's abuse on the patient's work. If the patient has just been referred by the employee assistance program because of a positive drug screen at the work site, this evaluation will most likely occur early in the assessment process. If, however, the patient's spouse or significant other has just left because of the substance abuse of the patient, it may not be possible to evaluate the impact of the abuse on the patient's work until much later in the assessment (sometimes not even until a subsequent session). Finally, if the patient presents because he or she has just been arrested for driving while intoxicated for the third time, the patient may be quite capable of complying with a highly structured, research-style interview. In the real world of daily clinical practice, patients present in all these ways and many more. The challenge, again, is to balance the need for structured data for outcomes management with the need for flexibility for good clinical practice. We have allowed the clinician to exercise his or her clinical judgment as to the timing of the specific area of the patient's life to be evaluated and provided a small number of quantifiable, structured items within each area to be investigated when it is the right time. In the example of the patient whose spouse has just left, the interview might proceed as follows: "Now, we've talked a lot about how your husband has just left you, and we will return to this later, but right now I'd like to look at how your drinking has affected other areas of your life, for example, your work. Can you tell me how many days you've missed from work in the last 60 days because of your drinking?" The patient gives a number; this number can be scaled, aggregated, and, most importantly, eventually compared with the number given 6 or 12 months later after treatment in response to the same question.

By balancing the structure required for methodologically sound outcomes evaluation with the flexibility required to minimize administrative burden on both patients and clinicians, we have been successful at engineering the outcomes management initiative into the routine of our organization. Currently, we collect structured baseline data about 14 clinical and functional outcome domains on every substance abuse patient treated at every one of our 40 or so substance abuse programs around the country. More importantly, we do so at no additional expense or burden to either the patient or the clinician. These thousands of baseline assessments are entered into a pretest outcomes database within our larger relational database. They are later combined with 6- and 12-month follow-up data to generate a delta (pretest – posttest = measured change).

At this point in the process, we enter the third stage of the journey toward accountability and improvability, which I call the analytical stage. For outcomes management, it is not enough to generate sound data about areas of a patient's life to be monitored on a routine and ongoing basis. These data also must be subjected to appropriate statistical analysis to be turned into meaningful information that correctly identifies opportunities for improvement. A good example of this is the need for case-mix adjustment of the data to understand treatment effect. Put simply, each patient brings strengths and weaknesses to treatment that in and of themselves can account for a significant proportion of that patient's improvement after treatment. If these strengths and weaknesses are not entered into the analysis of the outcomes data, any given treatment might be incorrectly evaluated. Examples include such simple case-mix adjusters as age and sex, which, along with diagnosis, form the basis for diagnosis-related groups. In psychiatry, however, we must always remember that these explain little of the variance in utilization of resources or treatment effect because if they did, psychiatry and substance abuse would have been subjected to prospective reimbursement in the early 1980s, when diagnosis-related groups were first introduced for medical-surgical care under Medicare. Perhaps a better example for behavioral care is the need to evaluate such case-mix areas as past treatment response and motivation to better understand differential treatment response. No knowledgeable mental health or substance abuse clinician would believe that an unmotivated patient has the same chance for a successful outcome as a motivated one; it only makes sense, then, as we attempt to understand what treatments work and which do not that we adjust for such factors in our analyses.

A good example of the importance of such case-mix data exists within our current outcomes management efforts at MCC. Using the case-mix data available and our baseline substance abuse assessments, we have been able to identify with a high degree of statistical certainty certain types of patients who are at high risk for not following through on treatment. We are currently sharing these profiles with our substance abuse clinicians in selected sites to allow them to identify these patients proactively. This "early warning" will in turn allow our clinicians to deploy specialized interventions designed to increase the patients' awareness of the need to follow through and actually engage in treatment.

This example in turn brings us to the last and, in many ways, the most challenging of the stages in our journey toward becoming an accountable and improvable delivery system in mental health and substance abuse care. This final stage I call the behavioral stage. It involves mastering the psychological and educational challenges of getting clinicians and others to change their behaviors based on the reasoned analysis of sound data. Such change, after all, has to be the ultimate goal of the journey because it is only through changing practice patterns and clinical programs that our various stakeholders, be they patients, payers, or policymakers, will begin to reap benefits of receiving care from such an accountable, improvable delivery system. In the end, the appreciation of the value of such an approach will be based not just on the financial results achieved but, more importantly, on the clinical results. It is only through such an approach that we as clinicians can guarantee that the quality of our work will be appreciated by nonclinicians and its value will be both proved and, more importantly, improved over time.

In looking back over the journey to date, I see how much has been learned. If I had to summarize this learning for those who choose to follow this same path, I would do so as outlined in the following discussions:

Define the Purpose and Scope of the Outcomes Initiative

It is extremely important for an organization to fully and clearly understand and agree on the ultimate purpose of any outcomes initiative. At one extreme lies the simple outcomes study, designed to answer simple questions such as Do our patients' symptoms get better under our care? I call this a simple question because it involves only pre- and posttest data collection along a small set of clinical domains, with no need for case-mix adjustment or ongoing follow-up. At the other extreme lies the fully developed outcomes management system (such as the one at MCC), designed to answer more complicated questions such as What patient characteristics are highly predictive of significant and positive changes in both clinical symptoms and a range of functional outcomes? or What treatment delivers the most cost-effective results for patients with certain characteristics, and can it be made even more cost-effective? These questions involve collecting and analyzing sophisticated clinical data, as well as developing appropriate ongoing administrative support.

Identify the Data Elements and Processes Required to Meet the Program Goals

When the questions to be addressed are specified, it is essential to identify the data elements needed to answer them. For simpler questions and small-scale studies, standard instruments, with proven reliability and validity, focusing on symptoms and/or functioning can be employed. For more sophisticated questions and programs, designed to serve as clinical quality improvement efforts, more detailed information about patient and treatment characteristics must be collected and available for analysis.

Integrate the Collection and Analysis of the Required Data Into Existing or Improved Clinical Processes

Whenever possible, the data required for outcomes analysis should be collected and integrated into the normal clinical work flows of the organization, such as registration and assessment. Avoid wherever possible duplicative or wasteful extra work for either the patient or the clinician. Equally important is establishing a routine process for distributing the results of these efforts throughout the organization.

Generate a Culture Within the Organization That Looks to Outcomes Data to Guide Action

Merely distributing the results of these outcomes efforts is not enough. Managers and clinicians must look to clinical outcomes data to guide clinical decision making. We must use information about the clinical and functional results of our efforts to counter otherwise simplistic and financially driven decisions about what constitutes appropriate care. It is only through such efforts that we will ultimately achieve our goal of managing care, not just dollars.

References

Bartlett J: Practice guidelines and outcomes management: future roles for psychiatrists. Paper presented at the meeting of the American Psychiatric Association, New Roles for Psychiatrists in Organized Systems of Care, Raleigh-Durham, NC, October 21–23, 1994a

Bartlett J: Practice guidelines: the managed care view, in Allies and Adversaries: The Impact of Managed Care on Mental Health Services. Edited by Schreter RK, Sharfstein SS, Schreter CA. Washington, DC, American Psychiatric Association, 1994b, pp 153–162

Berwick D, Godfrey A, Roessner J: Curing Health Care: New Strategies for Quality Improvement. San Francisco, CA, Jossey-Bass, 1990

Donabedian A: Exploration in Quality Assessment and Monitoring. Ann Arbor, MI, Health Newsletter Press, 1980

Mosher L: Alternatives to psychiatric hospitalization. N Engl J Med 309:79–80, 1983

Pothoff S, Kane R, Bartlett J, et al: Developing a managed care clinical information system to assess outcomes of substance abuse treatment. Clinical Performance and Quality Health Care 2:148–153, 1994

18 Restructuring for Survival: The Sheppard Pratt Transformation

Steven S. Sharfstein, M.D., M.P.A.
John J. Kent Jr., J.D.

In 1853, the Maryland legislature chartered "The Sheppard Asylum." The first patient was admitted in 1891. Just before that admission, the institution was renamed "The Sheppard and Enoch Pratt Hospital." Almost exactly 100 years later, the institution is being transformed into "The Sheppard Pratt Health System." This is the story of this last transformation, which continues to take place.

Historical Context

Moses Sheppard was a successful businessman and a prominent member of the Friends Meeting in Baltimore. In his latter years, he devoted himself to the public good. At one time, he was named warden for the city's poor, and he was a founder of the American Colonialist Society, an abolitionist organization devoted to the education of freed slaves, the sponsorship of their return to Africa, and the founding of a republic in Liberia. In the mid-1840s, he met Dorothea Dix. Miss Dix was a former Sunday school teacher from Cambridge, Massachusetts, who was just beginning her campaign for humane treatment for the "insane," as the mentally ill of the era were called. She had come to Maryland to investigate the plight of the insane who were mostly warehoused in almshouses or poor houses, as well as prisons. She wrote her "memorial," as her reports were called, and presented it to the General Assembly of Maryland in 1849, when Moses Sheppard was a prominent legislator. The following is an excerpt from that memorial:

> I have glanced at the inefficiency and cruelty of a poor house, imprisoned residence for the epileptic and the maniac. In imagination for a short time, place yourselves in their stead. Enter the horrid, noisome cell. Invest yourself with the fowl, tattered garments which scantily serve the purposes of decent covering. Caste yourself upon the loathsome pile of filthy straw. Find companionship in your own cries and groans or in the wailings and gibberings of wretches miserable like yourselves. Call for help and release for blessed words of soothing, and kind offices of care until the dull walls weary in sending you back the echo of your moans. Then if your self possession is not overwhelmed under the imagined miseries of what are the actual distresses of the insane, return to the consciousness of your sound intellectual health and answer, if you will, no longer refuse or delay to make adequate appropriation for the establishment of a hospital for the care and cure of those who are deprived of the use of their reasoning faculties.

Moses Sheppard was deeply moved by her appeal and became a key sponsor of this legislation, which established the first public mental hospital in Maryland. Miss Dix went on to similarly petition the legislatures in 18 states and personally led to the founding of some 22 state mental hospitals over the next two decades.

Moses Sheppard went to visit the York Retreat, a prominent Quaker institution in York, England, and on his return, in the late 1840s, determined to found an asylum under the private auspices first for members of the Society of Friends and then for others who could pay the fees, as well as all citizens who needed quality care and treatment. He wanted his institution to "lead the way" and "to combine every feature that science and experience might indicate as requisite or desirable to minister to the greatest possible advantage to the patient" (Forbush 1968, p. 228). So the Sheppard Asylum was chartered in 1853, and construction began after Moses Sheppard's death in 1857, utilizing as per the instructions in his will only the interest but not the principal in his bequest of approximately half a million dollars.

It was another 34 years before Sheppard opened its doors to its first patient. The interest from the bequest on an annual basis was not considerable, and the Civil War intervened. Because of the many delays in the construction of the Sheppard Asylum, there was a saying in Baltimore: "I'll get to it when Sheppard's finished." (Today, that statement is coming back into vogue.) Finally, it was ready for patients in 1890 but needed another gift for enough funds to hire staff. Enoch Pratt, another prominent Baltimore businessman, was approached, and he agreed to make a very generous bequest on the condition that his full name be inserted into the title of the institution; the trustees decided to move toward the modern term *hospital,* so the Sheppard Asylum was renamed The Sheppard and Enoch Pratt Hospital.

From the very beginning, The Sheppard and Enoch Pratt Hospital focused on inpatient care, was a long-term residence for patients with serious mental disorders, and functioned as a tertiary treatment center not only in Maryland but also regionally and nationally. Occupational therapy was the mainstay of treatment, and psychotherapy and psychoanalysis were important elements of care and teaching for prominent psychoanalysts such as Harry Stack Sullivan, Lewis Hill, Lawrence Kubie, and others who worked at Sheppard Pratt. The directors of the hospital were long term. When Dr. Robert Gibson was appointed in 1963, he was the fourth director since the opening of the hospital in 1891; when Dr. Steven Sharfstein was appointed in 1992, he was only the fifth in 100 years of care. Long-term care and long-term directors went hand in hand.

Some Clinical and Financial Statistics: 1989–1994

Perhaps the best way to describe the massive changes that have taken place and continue to take place at Sheppard Pratt are captured in some key clinical and financial statistics of the years 1989–1994. In Table 18–1, the length of stay, both means and medians, and the occupancy as well as admissions are portrayed.

In 1989, the last year of the "old" Sheppard Pratt Hospital with its focus on long-term inpatient care, the average length of stay for all patients was 70 days and for children and adolescents,

Table 18–1. Sheppard Pratt: 322-bed not-for-profit hospital

	1989	1992	1993	1994
Occupancy (%)	92	65	60	55
Average length of stay (days)	70	32	17	16
Median length of stay (days)	33	21	11	9
Child and adolescent average length of stay (days)	110	55	28	20
Child and adolescent median length of stay (days)	50	30	19	9
Bottom line	Positive	Negative	Break even	Positive

110 days. Occupancy in the 322-bed hospital averaged 92%. This occupancy had been consistent for more than 10 years, and Sheppard Pratt never experienced a year in which its financial bottom line was not in the black.

In 1993, the average length of stay hospital-wide had slipped to 17 days and occupancy to 60%. More than 100 beds had been closed during that year. Substantial downsizing of staff, clinical and administrative, occurred with a reduction in expenditures, and growth of inpatient alternatives accelerated with the opening of six new day treatment programs, satellite clinics and group homes, mobile treatment and home treatment, and the first at-risk subcapitated contract with the Kaiser Permanente health maintenance organization. The bottom line was "break even"; in fact, there was a small loss in operations, but this followed a year in which there had been a substantial loss as occupancy decreased dramatically in the face of managed care–driven reductions in length of stay. In 1994, average length of stay continued to decline to approximately 2 weeks. Occupancy had slipped further to 55% with some further closing of beds, but additional outpatient day programs were initiated, and the bottom line is now comfortably in the black. The Sheppard Pratt Hospital during 1992 through 1994 transformed and reinvented itself into the Sheppard Pratt Health System. There was a new mission, a new organizational structure was created, different financial incentives were created through the practice plan, and strategic directions were set to cope with and adapt to the radical restructuring of the financing of medical and psychiatric care that will continue to occur in this country for the foreseeable future.

The New Sheppard Mission

In the fall of 1992, a process was initiated to develop a new mission for the Sheppard Pratt Health System consistent with the evolving structure that had been put together to be responsive to the new paradigms of care delivery for patients with mental illness and substance abuse and to cut administrative costs.

The process of developing this mission involved more than 100 individuals who are employees, patients and family members, clinicians and nonclinicians, trustees, and consumer advocates. The mission statement was written to be fairly broad, and then a vision statement and strategic intent were developed to become more focused and specific. Ten guiding principles also were developed so that staff could begin to identify with the new mission of the Sheppard Pratt Health System. The mission, vision, and strategic intent statements and the 10 guiding principles were finalized in December 1992.

The *mission* statement reads as follows:

> The Sheppard and Enoch Pratt Health System is dedicated to innovation and excellence in the delivery of behavioral health, mental illness and addiction services. We will strive to help people enhance and restore their ability to function and improve their quality of life. We will continue our over 100-year tradition of superior treatment while advancing community presence, advocacy, education and research.

This statement was intended to be broad, emphasizing our connection with the past excellence of Sheppard Pratt but pointing to the future.

The *vision* statement reads as follows:

> The Sheppard and Enoch Pratt Health System will be the leader in providing quality services by offering a cost-effective continuum of care to all sectors of the population without regard to race, religion, color, national origin, sex, age, or disability.

In the vision statement, the concepts of cost-effectiveness and continuum of care and accessibility are introduced, which are critical in the development of a comprehensive care delivery system.

The *strategic intent* statement reads as follows:

> The Sheppard and Enoch Pratt Health System will achieve its mission by developing an integrated service delivery sys-

tem located throughout the Baltimore-D.C. region to meet
the needs of all of our customers.

In the strategic intent statement, the concept of an integrated
service delivery system and the primary area of focus for Sheppard Pratt are identified and, for the first time, the word *customers* is introduced.

To bring concepts emanating from the market and business
into health care is an important task for clinicians for whom
these notions are foreign and sometimes difficult to understand
or to tolerate. Many physicians went to medical school to avoid
going into business and always assumed the business of medicine would be a minor part of their practice career. However, in
the past few years, market forces have been introduced that dramatically change the paradigms for the delivery of treatment.
"Customer service" is an important philosophical underpinning
of any successful business. Customers are not only people who
buy the goods and services, but also people who help guide
those decisions and who help produce the product—the so-
called internal customers. Health care customers include patients and families, third and fourth parties, employers (as well
as government) who pay the bills, and internal customers to the
health care industry that include referrers and employed staff.

The 10 guiding principles for the new Sheppard Pratt Health
System are posted strategically throughout the various facilities
now forming the Sheppard Pratt Health System and read as
follows:

QUALITY: We will continuously improve all aspects of our
work. We will be primarily responsive to the needs of our
patients and clients as well as other customers—payers,
families, referrers, and staff. We will meet professional
standards in our field. We will strive to provide the highest
level of clinical care based on state-of-the-art treatment.

CARING: We will provide services with compassion and
with sensitivity to all of the needs of our patients and families.

CHARITY CARE: We will strive to provide financial assistance to individuals and families in need.

VALUE: We will deliver cost-effective and appropriately priced services to our customers.

INNOVATION: We will use the talent of staff and the latest scientific technology to create a model health care system.

COMMUNITY PRESENCE: We will deliver services in public/private partnerships through local and national education and advocacy.

LEARNING ENVIRONMENT: We will support a spirit of inquiry throughout the Health System and provide innovative teaching and research programs.

EMPOWERMENT: We will encourage independent decision making and the use of creativity to reach our goals.

CULTURAL DIVERSITY: We will deliver services to patients and clients without regard to race, religion, color, national origin, sex, age, or disability. We will view the cultural diversity of our staff as an asset to the system and will promote the recruitment of minority employees.

INTEGRITY: In all the above, we will uphold the highest standard of ethical, honest and forthright behavior.

Several of these principles are particularly important in terms of the special aspects of the Sheppard Pratt Health System. These special aspects include the emphasis on quality; the learning environment for adults and children and adolescents that is promoted by our accredited residency training programs; our other training efforts in psychology, social work, nursing, and pastoral counseling; and Sheppard Pratt's Quaker heritage, which emphasizes charity, community presence, cultural diversity, and integrity.

The mission statement was accompanied by a radical restructuring of the Sheppard system from a traditional hospital into service lines.

Service Lines

As mentioned earlier, the Sheppard Pratt Hospital has been a traditional, long-term inpatient treatment program—a service for which insurance companies reimbursed. Ambulatory programs were developed in response to the public sector expectations as well as the needs of the residency training program. Until recent years, ambulatory programs were not intended to be major contributors to the financial success of the organization. The health system has now been structured to provide for continuity of care, vertical integration, and alternatives to the inpatient bed. The service lines concept was developed in the search for an effective means to provide continuity of care to general and subspecialty patients and to provide quality care while meeting the expectations of external market forces for a competitively priced service.

Service lines then were developed to provide for a logical grouping of subspecialty services that promote access and continuity of care and have an identifiable external market. They were developed as a rationale-planning management unit, each with a clearly defined mission related to the superordinate health system mission, with an emphasis on responsiveness to changing needs of customers. Demonstrable positive outcomes for patients treated within the service line are an important component, with an emphasis on quality improvement.

This decentralized organization of services is required to focus in a rapid way on changing market forces and is expected to produce a positive bottom line. Although Sheppard Pratt is a "not-for-profit" institution, it has been emphasized that we are also "not for loss." Some of the service lines that are publicly funded are not able to generate a profit; however, these are expected to break even and make a contribution to overhead. This definition of service lines makes them "semiautonomous" business units because the key budgetary decisions, based on timely financial analysis, would be made by the service line managers.

Service line management then is both an externally driven strategy to capture market share and an internally driven strategy to operate more efficiently and effectively.

Eight service lines were initially developed at Sheppard Pratt. The first grouping is based on age. The *Child and Adolescent Service Line,* which has always had an identifiable inpatient program, was expanded to include day treatment, including a fully accredited special school, K–12, outpatient services, residential care for children and adolescents, home visits, and other targeted educational services aimed at children and adolescents. At the other end of the age spectrum, the *Geriatric Service Line,* was created to focus on the clinical needs of the elderly, including an expanded geriatric inpatient unit, psychogeriatric day treatment on and off campus, outpatient services, and outreach to nursing homes and life-care communities. The *General Adult Service Line,* with an emphasis on acute managed mental health care, constitutes the third age-related service line and includes inpatient care, day treatment, outpatient services, and residential and group home services. Carved out from this age-related set of service lines are three subspecialty areas. The first is the *Chemical Dependency Service Line,* with a dual-diagnosis inpatient unit, day treatment, intensive outpatient as well as evening care, outreach into the community, and educational programs. The *Dissociative Disorders Service Line* is a small program with a national referral base and includes an inpatient unit, a day treatment program, and some outpatient services and emphasizes the treatment of posttraumatic stress disorders, dissociative disorders, and dissociative identity disorder. The final subspecialty service line, initially called *Severely and Persistently Ill* and then changed to *Community Mental Health and Rehabilitation Service Line,* emphasizes the care of the seriously and chronically ill patient group and the commitment of Sheppard Pratt to community mental health. With public grants,

Sheppard Pratt provides a full continuum of treatment and psychosocial rehabilitation services in several areas of Baltimore County, as well as housing for a large group of patients with chronic schizophrenia and other chronic psychotic disorders. A quarterway house group home on the grounds of Sheppard and an inpatient program round out this particular service line. This service line is an example of public/private partnerships that are possible in this era of health care reform.

The two remaining service lines are the *Satellite Network Service Line* and *Preferred Resources.* The Satellite Network Service Line is a small management team that helps the other service lines get off the campus of Sheppard Pratt and develop satellite clinics, day programs, and group homes, as well as relationships with general hospitals, in the greater Maryland area. This service line has been developed in relation to our major strategic effort to become a comprehensive, regionally based mental health service delivery system. Preferred Resources provides employee assistance services, mostly in Maryland but also throughout the country. Related managed behavioral health care is part of this initiative, and it is through this initiative that Sheppard Pratt was able to compete and win a subcapitated at-risk contract with Kaiser Permanente to deliver comprehensive mental health and substance abuse services to 33,000 Kaiser Permanente enrollees in Maryland.

In the process of putting together vertically integrated service lines, hospital departmental structure was radically altered. All nurses are now budgeted in and report to their respective service line; however, the nursing department retains responsibility for credentialing, continuing education, and quality assurance activity. The same is true for social work, rehabilitation therapy, psychology, and psychiatry. A new position, director of clinical services, was created. The former director of nursing filled this position and is responsible for all the centralized clinical services mentioned, as well as pharmacy and the department of medicine. Other centralized services include the finance division and general support services division, which maintains the 105-acre campus in Towson and the various satellite clinics.

Each of the service lines has a different staffing pattern, depending on the program and target population, and there is the expectation that staff will flexibly move along the continuum of care depending on demand and need with the goal of continuity of care for patients. To understand how this works, a brief description of a changed economic incentive plan for psychiatrists and psychologists is appropriate.

New Economic Incentives for Clinicians

Coinciding with the restructuring of Sheppard into service lines was a new system for psychiatrists, psychologists, and some social workers, emphasizing patient care and productivity and providing an opportunity for compensation beyond the expected number of patient encounters for clinicians. This system employs the concept of a "relative value unit" (RVU) system of payment.

Practice Plan

The RVU system was instituted in 1992. Before then, physicians and psychologists were salaried by the practice plan as either full- or part-time employees. Within their contract was an estimate of the amount of clinical work expected as well as other activities, including teaching, administration, and research. These expectations, which were negotiated annually, assumed that clinicians would continue at Sheppard Pratt as long as they wished to.

This all changed dramatically in 1992 with the reorganization and restructuring. Every clinician was expected to sign a 1-year contract, and clinical expectations were restructured in terms of annual productivity, which was based on RVUs. A compensation committee was formed to develop a menu of RVUs for clinical services provided. This menu, which is continuously revised, is provided in Table 18–2.

Table 18–2. Relative value unit schedule

Clinical service	RVU
A. Inpatient	
1. Admissions	1.74
2. Primary care/day	0.70
3. Attending (PGY I,II)/day	0.35
4. Attending (PGY IV)/day	0.28
5. Attending + medical management (LCSW)/day	0.40
6. Attending + medical management (PD)/day	0.40
7. Attending/admissions (PGY, PD)	0.44
8. Medical management/day	0.17
9. Weekend attending/patient	0.29
B. Outpatient: adult	
1. Intake	2.15
2. Individual 30 min/visit	0.71
3. Individual up to 40 min/visit	1.07
4. Individual 41–60 min/visit	1.43
5. Individual 90 min/visit	2.15
6. Individual 120 min/visit	2.87
7. Group visit/patient (90 min):	
sessions 1–4	1.00
sessions 5 +	0.71
8. Group visit/patient (60 min)	0.47
9. Medication checks/visit	0.57
C. Outpatient: child and adolescent	
1. Intake	3.80
2. Individual 30 min/visit	0.77
3. Individual up to 40 min/visit	1.14
4. Individual 41–60 min/visit	1.52
5. Individual 90 min/visit	2.28
6. Individual 120 min/visit	3.04
7. Group visit/patient (90 min):	
sessions 1–4	1.00
sessions 5 +	0.77
8. Group visit/patient (60 min)	0.51
9. Medication checks/visit	0.57
D. Consultations	1.75
E. Peer review panel	2.33
F. Panels	hour for hour
Certification hearings	
Appeals hearings	
Administrative review determinators hearings	

Note. RVU = relative value unit. Time (hours) × work intensity (acuity of patient, collateral contacts needed, stress on the clinician) × value to health system (e.g., mission, profitability). Work intensity and value are arrived at through a process of consensus by the clinicians.

Total RVU expectations are negotiated with each clinician and contracted for each year. This base pay is guaranteed at 100% of total hours contracted. In the early implementation of this system, management reserved 20% of pay if RVU targets were not met. It was found in implementation that this was unnecessary and a morale problem for clinicians, especially considering the annual renegotiation of contracts and the possibility either to cut back time or terminate employees.

A bonus can be earned if clinicians go beyond their negotiated RVUs. The over-caseload pay kicks in when 100% of productivity expectations have been met. This is done at a flat rate per RVU rather than as a multiple of the hourly rate.

In the first year of the implementation of this program, over-caseload payments approached $500,000. In the second year, these payments increased to more than $700,000. During the same time period, many more patients were treated within the Sheppard Pratt Health System, and fewer clinicians were employed.

This system of productivity and over-caseload compensation has made possible a number of flexible innovations, including clinician coverage throughout the continuum of care, clinician coverage on nights and weekends, cross-coverage during illness and vacation, and other ways for clinicians to continue to "earn RVUs."

A downside to this approach has been a reduction in the willingness of clinicians to participate in activities for which there is no RVU reimbursement. Many of these goodwill or marketing activities are important to the health system, and clinicians need extra encouragement to spend other hours on some of these activities. Time spent on the telephone with utilization reviewers, referrers, and others also does not get RVU reimbursement. Another potential problem for the system is what to do when more activity is reimbursed on a capitated rather than a retrospective fee-for-service basis. The RVU system is predicated on fee-for-service reimbursement. Capitation implies less rather than more, and perhaps the system needs to be revised so that clinicians get a "bundled" RVU for an entire episode of care and assume some risk for treating the patient within that particular RVU credit. As more patients come in through prospective payment, other salary arrangements may need to be developed.

The RVU system has been constructed on the basis of service rendered rather than amount or source of payment. As such, the system cross-subsidizes Medicaid and self-pay patients who cannot afford the physician's fees. This issue does create some stress within the overall salary structure; however, our reimbursement system attempts to encourage that one mode of practice will be provided regardless of source of payment.

The numbers of patients seen by Sheppard clinicians have multiplied, and income has grown. Often clinicians complain about this system, but when presented with alternatives that would eliminate some of the positives such as over-caseload, they have decided to make continuous improvements to the current RVU system. It is indeed a collaborative venture with a great deal of input from the practice plan clinicians all along the way.

Strategic Directions

More critical than the mission statement are the four strategic directions that guide each service line within the health system. These four directions were developed during an intense 2-day strategic planning retreat with staff and trustees. They guide the development of budget, new programs, and everyday activities for clinicians and administrators within the health system.

The first strategic direction is to reduce cost per episode of illness. This strategic direction addresses the fundamental shift in mental health care and its financing from intensive and expensive care for a few patients to cost-efficient and cost-effective care for many. The shift away from long-term psychiatric hospitalization is an example of this. It is clear that those mental health care providers that can reduce their costs and treat those in need within a large population group will survive and grow. The high-cost intensive treatment providers, however, will find themselves increasingly isolated as health reform continues to change the clinical and economic incentives.

Sheppard Pratt, like many other private psychiatric hospitals, has traditionally been a high-cost provider. As a tertiary care referral center, Sheppard accepts patients who are treatment resistant, and the clinical philosophy has been to develop ambitious treatment goals emphasizing costly inpatient care. Reducing our costs on an episode-of-illness basis will allow Sheppard to compete with managed private and public systems of care now and in the future.

Using alternatives to the inpatient setting, retraining staff on new modes of practice, using staff more efficiently and effectively throughout the continuum of care, and reducing our overhead or indirect costs are all elements of this cost reduction strategy.

The second strategic direction is to expand prospective payment, sharing risk and capitation. This strategic direction addresses the fact that the world is moving in the direction of prospective payment and capitation. The contrast between prospective payment and fee-for-service retrospective reimbursement is profound. Health maintenance organizations are growing. Relationships with these organizations are essential, as is developing other strategies to managed care.

Currently, Sheppard manages almost 40,000 "lives," mostly through the Kaiser Permanente carve-out subcapitated contract for mental health and substance abuse services. This contract requires a specific investment in case management, gatekeeping, information systems, and quality or outcome measures to develop the best efficiency and effectiveness for this particular population. Sheppard's experience with community mental health is quite helpful, and the service lines that focus on alternatives to inpatient care are quite critical. Hospital diversion programs such as crisis home-based or emergency room care become important within this strategic direction as well.

The third strategic direction is to expand noninpatient services throughout the metropolitan region. Sheppard Pratt recognized that it had to move off its 105-acre campus and become a primary and secondary care provider near the homes of the people we treat. Satellite clinics, day hospitals, residential groups, contracts with general hospital psychiatric units, and mobile treatment are all elements of this strategy. Public sector contracts, which expand our presence throughout the state, as well as our public/private partnerships, are also elements of this strategic direction. With these expansions, we now can bid on population-based or capitated contracts and achieve our objectives, as well as our second strategic direction.

The fourth strategic direction is to develop alliances and potential joint ventures. It is quite clear that despite its size, Sheppard Pratt is not big enough to go it alone. Partnerships, joint ventures, and even mergers with compatible health and mental health systems are quite likely. Sheppard Pratt has developed a close relationship with a general hospital contiguous to its property, the Greater Baltimore Medical Center. Many joint projects have evolved over the last several years, including projects that merge the campuses. This general hospital has taken the lead in developing its own health network throughout the state. Other partnerships or joint ventures with managed care delivery systems are also likely. The short-range cost efficiencies will help achieve the first strategic direction, and the long-range positioning and market share will help achieve the second and third strategic directions.

These four strategic directions help inform our service line managers as they pick and choose, within constrained budgets, opportunities for new programs and new clinical services.

Conclusion

Crisis has a tendency to focus one's attention. The 19th-century Sheppard Asylum and the 20th-century Sheppard and Enoch Pratt Hospital are emerging into the 21st century as The Sheppard Pratt Health System. This system brings clinical and administrative concepts of community mental health developed in the public sector to bear in the private not-for-profit comprehensive delivery system that defines Sheppard Pratt. Awareness of costs, application of the most efficacious diagnosis and treatment, and responsiveness to customers, broadly defined, are all hallmarks of this new Sheppard Pratt. Clinicians are working harder and seeing more patients for longer hours to achieve their own personal compensation goals. In the community, people look to Sheppard Pratt as a high-quality community provider. As the world moves toward prospective payment and capitation, Sheppard Pratt is poised to deliver population-based treatment and prevention as it readies itself for the next 100 years of quality care.

Reference

Forbush B: Moses Sheppard: Quaker Philanthropist of Baltimore. Philadelphia, PA, JB Lippincott, 1968

19 Training Residents in the Era of Managed Care

Donald R. Ross, M.D.

We currently are on the cusp of a new era of mental health care. Managed care is dominating the field and forcing a new cost consciousness and different, more efficient models of care. We cannot be clear where things will stabilize, but we have a vertiginous sense of being sucked toward it at an accelerating pace. What are the challenges in training future psychiatrists as we face the "era of managed care" (which may be a transitional "era" into the new order of things)? If we do not adequately adjust our educational approaches now to face today's challenges, we will be hopelessly disoriented 5 or 10 years from now as the new era of mental health care becomes more clearly defined and firmly established.

The Basic Problem

The basic problem we face training psychiatric residents in the era of managed care is that we are confused about our identity as psychiatrists. Managed care has upset the apple cart. We were used to a system controlled by psychiatrists (as clinicians) where patients were either inpatients or outpatients. Now we face a system controlled by administrators (who may be psychiatrists in an administrative role) where clinical responsibility is diffuse and patients can be anywhere in a broad continuum of care. To the extent we are unsure of our role in this new arrangement, we lose our clarity of vision in training our residents.

I believe we need to end this confusion as quickly as we can. The first and most important task we face in accomplishing this is to find and reestablish our moral center. We need to be clear about the fundamental principles that guide the profession of medicine and psychiatry and the critical principles that inform the teaching of residents.

Training future psychiatrists is not nearly as clear and straightforward as training is for the young osprey I saw winging out to sea with his father. I was witness to a hunting lesson. The young osprey was being taught how to hover in the face of the salt spray, how to fight the powerful crosswinds, how to spot the shadow of a fish, and how to fold his wings and experience that moment of falling, faster and faster, on the very edge of control, diving through the air to pierce the water, snare the fish, and rise triumphantly from the water with powerful strokes of his water-soaked wings. When he got it right (on his third try), I imagined it must have been the defining moment for the young raptor. It was all of a whole. He knew who he was and what his life's work was. His father taught it to him, he learned it, and someday he will teach it to his fledgling.

Like the osprey, we need a clear vision of who we are and what our life work is so that we too can confidently teach our fledglings. Cormac McCarthy's (1994) play, *The Stonemason*, makes this point even more clear. A stonemason learns the craft from a master stonemason by laying stone and watching stone being laid. This is not armchair knowledge, and if it is, it is useless. The stonemason lifts stones of different shapes and weight, feels each stone in his or her hands, balances it, imagines its place in the structure. Day after day of working with stone teaches the stonemason an intimacy with the force of gravity, with that irresistible, irreducible force that dominates the work. The stonemason learns how a properly laid hearth creates the conditions for a properly laid wall. The wall is straight and holds against the elements and over time. Quality control involves the simplest and most elegant of instruments, the plumb line, a weight on a string that is pulled down toward earth by gravity until it rests straight, taut, and true.

Where is our plumb line? What are the forces that make up the essential aspect of our work, the forces that might be analogous to gravity for the stonemason? We may have no animal instinct, no gravity, no plumb line per se, but we need to identify the deep guiding principles that we do have. These principles will tug at our shoulder, move us in the right direction even as we suffer the disorientation of these historical changes in psychiatry. If we do not ground ourselves in these principles, we are certainly lost and have nothing to teach anyone.

Our second task is to come to grips with the fact that the era of managed care is here for the foreseeable future. We need to acknowledge that this represents a change of historical magnitude. We need to understand what this means for medicine, psychiatry, and the training of psychiatric residents. We must adapt to the new managed care environment and try to have some say in shaping it.

Third, we need to understand *why* the era of managed care has put such a radical stress on us that we have questioned our very identity. What makes the changes we face so cataclysmic and the moment so historic? It is because the control of health care has changed hands. Now there is a competing value system based on bottom-line economics and cost containment that is trying to define our work. Physicians have lost control over the money in health care. Professional administrators control the money now. Whether we like this or not, whether we think it is a good idea or not, is irrelevant. It is a fact. Professional administrators run the health systems in which most psychiatric residency training programs are embedded. Administrators run the insurance companies and managed care companies controlling the money that the health system needs to survive. We have much less autonomy, much less self-determination, in this new environment.

Fourth, we need to realize we are in the midst of a very *fluid* historical moment. We are still struggling with how to shape the deeply personal realms of medicine and psychiatry now that administrators are running the show. There certainly is a lot at stake, most critically the quality of patient care and the definition of the physician's (and the psychiatrist's) professional identity. For example, the physician-patient relationship is in grave danger of losing its central position in the practice of medicine. The administrators are inclined to see the problems and opportunities in terms of populations of patients, systems of health care delivery, external quality assurance monitors, practice guidelines, and reduction of costs.

Needless to say, these are challenging conditions in which to train residents. If it is to be done well, psychiatrists and administrators need to agree on some fundamental values and goals in the delivery of mental health care, need to understand the elements that go into good training, and need to believe training psychiatrists is worthwhile.

The Core Values of Modern Psychiatry

I would propose that four core values should direct us into the future: 1) quality patient care, 2) sound economic policies and decisions, 3) academic integrity, and 4) a humanistic approach to treating patients and to training residents. Putting these four values together means that patients should get the best care we can offer them under the economic realities of today's marketplace. In the process of designing such care, we should carefully and honestly assess what we know about treating mental illness. In addition, we should give of ourselves in a caring and committed way, with respect for each other—patient, resident, and staff member. This last component costs nothing and often makes a tremendous difference in outcome and in job satisfaction.

Quality patient care is often thought to have an inverse relationship with economic resources. This is not necessarily true. For example, a 3-year hospitalization on a personality disorders unit for a patient with borderline personality disorder may not be better than twice-weekly outpatient psychotherapy for 5 years with intermittent brief hospitalizations when the patient becomes suicidal. In fact, an occasional extended one- or two-session focused therapy intervention with an open-door policy for return visits might be even better for certain patients with this configuration of symptoms and character traits. We still have a lot to learn about what constitutes effective treatment for many of our patients. We need well-designed outcome studies to guide us. But to assume that we should offer only the last option because it is cheapest is just as wrong as pushing the first option because we have a personality disorders unit to fill.

Quality patient care means a number of things. It means using all of our knowledge, gathered from our science and our collective experience in the art of psychiatry, in the service of the patient. It means working to restore the patient to the greatest possible health and functional capacity and to alleviate suffering. It means dedicating ourselves to our patients and our craft in a way that is deep and abiding. Over a lifetime of such dedicated work, it means developing a wisdom and humanitarian perspective that can be healing in and of itself. Providing quality patient care helps to define us as psychiatrists in ways similar to the life work of the osprey and the stonemason.

Quality patient care does not mean doing everything possible for each individual patient regardless of the cost in terms of money or suffering. It is not a personal crusade against death or mental illness. It is not a quest to be the idealized parent to the needy patient or the obsessionally complete attending physician to the extremely complicated patient. Quality care also is not the best compromise that can be reached in the face of economic limitations. Quality patient care is not the best educated guess in a benefit-to-risk-to-cost equation. In fact, quality care cannot be reliably attained from a single driving force. True quality patient care evolves out of three separate foci—the needs of the patient, the guiding principles of the profession of psychiatry (including the awareness of economic factors and the results of outcome studies), and personal motivations within the physician (sublimated motivations that led the physician to this calling). Being mindful of each of these and balancing them lead to quality patient care.

Every resident needs to train at an institution that is committed to quality patient care. There is no substitute for dedicated mentors and supervisors who have thoroughly identified with these values. This is necessary, but not sufficient for a good training program in today's managed care environment.

Education concerning *economic issues* also needs to play an integrated role in the training of psychiatric residents. Residents need to learn how to conceptualize an inpatient stay in terms that reflect the very expensive use of resources that it actually represents. The resident cannot in good conscience simply ask, "Would it make my life and the patient's life easier if I brought the patient into the hospital?" Instead, the resident must address the questions, "Does the patient require 24-hour nursing care?" and "What needs to be done in the hospital so that such intensive care is no longer necessary?"

At the moment, these are questions asked by the managed care reviewers. But these questions need to become incorporated into the natural questions psychiatrists and residents ask themselves before deciding on admitting a patient to the hospital. These questions need to be seen as part of the guiding principle of fiscal responsibility that needs to be part of the central value system of each new physician. The money question cannot remain a battle between administrators and clinicians. It needs to be cast in a broader light that takes into account the fact of our limited health care resources for an entire population of patients. Residents need to learn this set of values during their residency, to make it part of their identity as responsible physicians.

One important way this is learned is by designing the training program so that each resident gains experience in all sectors of the continuum of care. Residents who gain firsthand experience working in a day hospital will understand when it is preferable to admit a suicidal patient there instead of to the inpatient unit. Residents who work with a mobile treatment team will learn how to work with a chronic patient who has trouble staying on medication and thus prevent a relapse and hospitalization. Skillful use of the continuum of care will convince the resident that quality patient care and cost containment are often complementary processes.

One unfortunate trend in the battle between physicians and managed care companies has been the shortsighted notion that residents add cost to the care of the patient and therefore should not be involved in the care of the patient. There are no hard data to support the claim that residents add cost. In fact, the few controlled studies on this indicate that patients treated by residents have equal or shorter hospital stays compared with those treated by staff physicians (Buchwald et al. 1989; Udvarhelyi et al. 1990). The result of this battle has been an unnecessary and harmful animosity between residents and managed care reviewers. Through dialogue and mutual education, we have to promote involvement of residents with managed patient care. One way this has worked well has been with capitated contracts. Residents can provide quality care for the patient, save the health system money, and get the education they need concerning managed care and cost containment.

Finally, it is essential that residents get intensive training in brief focused psychotherapy. This cost-effective treatment approach is an essential part of the psychiatrist's therapeutic armamentarium today. Training in brief therapy is best done in a way that makes it clear that it is *not* a second-best option compared with long-term psychotherapy. I believe that long-term psychodynamic psychotherapy remains an important part of residency training. However, becoming a good long-term psychotherapist is *not* enough to prepare one to become a good short-term therapist. Residents need to learn certain attitudes, strategies, and techniques that are specific for brief focused therapy. To do this well, they need didactic instruction and supervision by faculty who are advocates of brief therapy and experts in this area.

Academic integrity is the third core value that residents need to absorb. The tension between quality patient care and economic restrictions is best addressed with an attitude of academic honesty. This involves gathering our knowledge, looking at it critically, and making decisions based on the conclusions we draw from the data. As a field, psychiatry has worked hard to describe and classify the varieties of mental disorders objectively. The result has been DSM-IV (American Psychiatric Association 1994a). We have also begun to develop treatment guidelines based on a critical review of our current knowledge base. Treatment guidelines for depression (American Psychiatric Association 1993b), eating disorders (American Psychiatric Association 1993a), and bipolar disorder (American Psychiatric Association 1994b) are already published. These guidelines are not "cookbook," but allow for well-thought-out variations. They also point the way to future research that will meaningfully study treatment outcomes.

The education of residents must occur in an environment that stimulates curiosity, therapeutic innovativeness, critical thinking and outcome studies. Residents should be fully indoctrinated into the process of gathering and critically evaluating our current base of knowledge. This is one part of an academic approach to psychiatry. Ongoing research is another key part of an academic environment. This research should address questions that will improve patient care and make it more cost-effective. Abandoning research because it is expensive is short sighted. However, it makes good sense to separate the funding for research from the funding for patient care so that academic institutions can properly compete with other mental health care systems for contracts to treat populations of patients.

Humanistic caring is the final principle we need to hold fast to and teach to our residents. We need to appreciate our patients' suffering, both objectively and empathically, if we are to be of help to them. Obviously, this is intimately connected to the other three values described: quality patient care, economic decisions that are responsive to cost containment, and commitment to academic honesty and research.

Dr. Francis Weld Peabody said, "the secret of the care of the patient is in caring for the patient" (Peabody 1927, p. 882). Unfortunately, medicine too often has forgotten this truth in its emphasis on better science and more effective technologies. Psychiatry has been slower than general medicine at losing the emphasis on the physician-patient relationship. With the advances in neuroscience and psychopharmacology, however, we are more frequently treating "neurotransmitter imbalances" instead of patients and closing the distance between ourselves and our medical colleagues.

Some administrators would take us a step further in this direction by limiting psychiatric interventions to diagnostic or psychopharmacological consultations. The biopsychosocial paradigm of human illness, which has been one of the great advances that psychiatry has offered the larger world of medicine, is in serious danger of fragmentation. Psychiatry is being offered the "bio" part alone in some mental health care systems. This would be a terrible loss to our professional identity, would make us less of a whole physician to our patients, and would result in a rapid deterioration in patient care. This is one area we still need to stand up and fight for when we see it in danger of being swept away by economic concerns.

Finally, humanistic values need to permeate the training experience itself. Residents can no longer be seen as cheap labor that can be exploited by the health system. There is a long tradition of working residents beyond healthy limits to toughen them to fatigue, human suffering, and dying patients. It not only toughens them, it makes them insensitive to their patients. There often has been an arrogance within the faculty of our academic medical institutions that has allowed residents to be treated as less than physicians, even less than people. This has been immortalized in the humorous classic, *House of God* (Shem 1981). Still, the experience of being an abused resident has never been funny, and it has no place in proper training today. If certain faculty members cannot understand that and change, then they should be dismissed. They should not be training our residents.

We want our residents to become practitioners who care about their patients, who take the time to listen to their concerns, and who are "customer-friendly" (which means little more than being a decent human being to another human being). We want our residents to become practitioners who work cooperatively and productively with other mental health professionals. All of this directly leads to better patient care. We need to model this humanistic attitude and behavior by treating our residents with respect and dignity. Abusive call schedules, excessive caseloads, and mindless scut work, on the one hand, and inadequate teaching and supervision, on the other, are ways that this abuse has been promulgated in the past. It should have no place in this new era.

Teaching the Core Values in a Psychiatric Residency Training Program: General Principles

The basic strategy to developing and maintaining a good psychiatric residency training program is simple. It involves three interrelated tasks: 1) recruit the best possible residents, 2) attract and retain the best possible faculty and keep them tightly attached to the residents, and 3) educate and form a solid working alliance with the administrators.

The first strategy is this: to have an excellent training program, have excellent residents. Recruitment is critical, especially in this climate of decreasing numbers of American medical school graduates entering psychiatry. If the program has excellent residents, and if they are happy with the quality of their training, they will recruit for you. Nothing compares to quality residents interviewing quality applicants and giving an honest and positive review of the training program.

Quality residents will make you work hard to satisfy their educational needs. But they will help you with that by providing energy and intellectual rigor to seminars and clinical work and by challenging and stimulating faculty. If you give residents the opportunity (through regular meetings and/or retreats), they will help you identify the weak points in the training program and help design improvements. Not only does this lead to a better educational program, but it also is a strong factor in building and maintaining a high morale. In so many ways, excellent residents are the first and foremost resource of a good training program.

The second strategy is to select, promote, and nurture the best possible faculty. These should be individuals who embody the core values discussed (quality patient care, economic awareness, academic honesty, and humanistic attitude). They should be inspiring teachers. The best faculty should be on the front lines teaching residents and medical students. The training director should put effort into understanding the unique gifts of each faculty member and then arrange that that faculty member has the opportunity to share those gifts with the residents. When the faculty see that they are appreciated by the residents and make a difference in the quality of the program, they become more closely identified with the mission of the residency training program. Besides creating a better program, the training director now also has natural allies in negotiations with the administration.

The volunteer faculty, who are often older, analytically oriented psychiatrists, present a unique challenge. These faculty members are often some of the most valuable teachers and supervisors for the residents. They are wise, thoughtful, and caring mentors and often inspire residents by providing models of how personal maturity leads to professional maturity in psychiatry. They have valuable perspectives on what is happening to psychiatry in this era of managed care. They are attuned to what psychiatry can lose if cost containment is pursued with single-minded purpose. Unfortunately, some of these faculty members feel strongly that we should take a decisive stand against the current changes. They may see the training director and the residents as natural allies in this fight and may exert significant pressure in that direction. This can intensify a split in the faculty that eventually demoralizes the residents they are supervising.

We have to help all our faculty understand the perspective of treating populations of patients cost-effectively so that they can align with change in good faith. We need to use their input to help structure specific changes. We have to get them interested in short-term psychotherapy and in applying dynamic principles to problems of medication noncompliance with patients who are not traditional psychotherapy patients.

The third general strategy for training residents in today's managed care environment involves working closely with the administrators. The ideal working relationship is one in which both the administrators and the clinicians (including the residents) feel respected and valued. When that happens, there is the freedom to collaborate on new approaches to mental health care delivery. This offers the possibility for providing quality care for more patients with the limited resources available. Any institution with such an advanced collaborative working relationship has a tremendous advantage over other competing institutions, both for attracting top-quality staff and for providing cost-effective and high-quality patient care. A continual adversarial relationship does little more than waste resources and demoralize everyone.

A corollary of this strategic goal is that the residency training program is always part of a larger health system. The health system is not in existence to support a training program; rather, the training program should work toward demonstrating its unequivocal value to the larger health system at every opportunity. This should not be hard to accomplish if it is a high-quality program. Residents bring life and vitality to a health system, attract top faculty and staff, provide onerous services such as overnight call, and demand quality care for patients. Often, the residents are the most sensitive barometer of the moral fidelity of the health system. If they are well trained, they will keep the clinicians and the administrators true to the four core values: quality patient care, cost consciousness, academic honesty, and a humanistic approach to the practice of medicine. Finally, the residents who graduate from a good training program form an important core of the full-time and volunteer faculty. They also are a critical part of the referral base to the hospital and other specialty areas within the health system.

Despite these obvious benefits to the health system, the residency training director and the residents themselves are wise to take nothing for granted. Residents are almost as costly as staff psychiatrists (if they are not exploited with excessive labor demands and are offered quality teaching and supervision). There is no room for a sense of entitled arrogance on the part of a good residency program. Instead, it should constantly work toward becoming increasingly invaluable to the larger health system of which it is a part.

A Specific Strategic Issue: The Role of Long-Term Psychotherapy Training and Personal Psychotherapy

One area that stirs up more controversy than any other is the role of long-term psychotherapy training for resident psychiatrists. Is long-term psychotherapy training worth the time and effort, given the fact that most patients in large health systems will receive psychotherapy from less costly mental health professionals? The role of the psychiatrist under managed care is often that of a diagnostician, a medical consultant and prescriber of medications, and a leader of a multidisciplinary treatment team. There may be some cases where the best and most cost-effective treatment involves a psychiatrist providing both the medical management and the psychotherapy for a particularly difficult patient. But this needs to be rare if the managed care arm of the health system is to do its job of keeping down costs.

Also, the vast majority of psychotherapy approved by managed care is focused, problem specific, and supportive in nature. Long-term, exploratory, psychoanalytically oriented psychotherapy is very limited in managed care systems.

Yet, often it is the values inherent in long-term psychodynamic psychotherapy—the power of the unconscious mind, the uniqueness of the individual patient, the healing potential of knowing a patient deeply within a caring relationship for an extended period—that have attracted psychiatric residents to this profession. Furthermore, a well-grounded understanding of psychodynamics is extremely helpful in working with patients (and staff) in all sorts of settings. It helps inform diagnostic interviewing, inpatient work, short-term psychotherapy, and medication management (especially compliance issues). A solid understanding of personality comes from psychodynamic training, and all patients have personalities that influence their illnesses and their treatment.

I would argue that a well-trained psychiatrist still needs a solid educational experience in long-term psychodynamic psychotherapy, even if the opportunities for incorporating this particular treatment modality into his or her daily professional life are much reduced or even nonexistent. A solid educational experience still requires adequate time devoted to treatment of at least a handful of long-term psychotherapy patients. These should include patients of both sexes and patients from both the healthier and the more ill ends of the spectrum. A good experience might be a neurotic college student with an anxiety disorder, a self-mutilating borderline patient, a chronically depressed mother of three young children, and a reclusive patient who hears voices in his or her head, has dissociated experiences, and has a history of childhood abuse. Working with a group of patients such as these once or twice a week for 1–2 years, with adequate individual supervision and appropriate course work, should provide the resident with an adequate immersion in psychodynamic psychotherapy.

Besides treating the patients, an additional focus should be on the countertransference reactions of the individual resident. A goal of this experience should be to develop a greater awareness of personal feelings and conflicts that arise in the treatment of particular types of patients or around particular issues or presentations. For example, it will be critically important that the psychiatric resident work through feelings about suicidal patients, demanding patients, withdrawn patients, angry patients, and so on. This is most meaningful when done in the context of an ongoing therapy relationship with the patient and an ongoing supervisory relationship with an experienced clinician.

What is the role of personal psychotherapy for residents? This is another thorny question. Personal therapy is personal, yet it is also an invaluable educational experience for psychiatrists. It helps one recognize previously unconscious conflicts that otherwise might be acted out to the detriment of the patient and the psychiatrist. It brings one in touch with sexual and aggressive wishes and anxieties that are frequently stirred up in work with patients. What role should it have in training psychiatric residents? How far should the training program go in supporting it? This becomes an even stickier issue as insurance coverage for personal therapy is now frequently limited to conditions where therapy is medically necessary and to treatment techniques that are problem focused and strictly time limited.

My recommendation is that personal therapy be a viable option for all residents who elect to undergo it. For most residents to afford therapy, there needs to be some subsidization either by the therapist or by the program. One approach is to develop a panel of therapists willing to see residents at a reduced rate. Another strategy is to establish a budget within the residency training program to provide some financial subsidy for residents in therapy. Moonlighting opportunities are also helpful, as long as they do not interfere with the education of the resident or the rules of the institution. Even with moonlighting, I feel that a minimum subsidy (either by a reduced fee or a "therapy allowance") should be 50% of once-a-week therapy sessions for at least 2 years. This amounts to a maximum of $5,000 granted to each resident who elects to undergo 2 years of personal therapy. I can think of no better investment in the resident's education. Waiting until residents can afford therapy on their own, when they become full-fledged practicing psychiatrists, is a mistake. Residency is a period when habits and ways of thinking (or defensively not thinking) are formed concerning critical problems in our work. I think training programs should send the message to residents that we encourage and support personal therapy for them. Supporting personal therapy for our residents makes it clear that we believe it has value beyond the purely medical alleviation of symptoms and that it has the potential to make them better psychiatrists. Under this system, insurance companies and managed care companies do not have to become involved, which further protects the confidentiality of the resident.

Finally, tangible support for personal therapy and for long-term psychodynamic psychotherapy training is a strong recruiting tool. If it is integrated into a well-rounded program, it will attract those residents most interested in integrating the exciting advances in the neurosciences with the mysteries of the human psyche as they manifest themselves in interpersonal relationships. The importance of this should not be underestimated. We are training psychiatrists who will practice for the next 30–40 years, a time span that will see tremendous changes in psychiatry. When all is said and done, the crucible of therapeutic change frequently requires a psychiatrist who is skilled, experienced, and at home in the intimacies of the physician-patient relationship.

References

American Psychiatric Association: Practice guideline for eating disorders. Am J Psychiatry 150:207–228, 1993a

American Psychiatric Association: Practice guideline for major depressive disorders in adults. Am J Psychiatry 150 (April suppl):1–26, 1993b

American Psychiatric Association: Diagnostic and Statistical Manual of Mental Disorders, 4th Edition. Washington, DC, American Psychiatric Association, 1994a

American Psychiatric Association: Practice guideline for the treatment of patients with bipolar disorder. Am J Psychiatry 151 (Dec suppl):1–36, 1994b

Buchwald D, Komaroff A, Cook EF, et al: Indirect costs for medical education. Arch Intern Med 149:765–768, 1989

McCarthy C: The Stonemason. Hopewell, NJ, Ecco Press, 1994

Peabody FW: The care of the patient. JAMA 88:877–882, 1927

Shem S: House of God. New York, Dell, 1981

Udvarhelyi I, Rosborough T, Lofgren RP, et al: Teaching status and resource use of patients with acute myocardial infarction: a new look at the indirect costs of graduate medical education. Am J Public Health 80:1095–1100, 1990

IV

Public Policy Issues
and the Continuum

20 Role of the Public Sector

Bernard S. Arons, M.D.
Sandra Raynes Weiss

Mental illness significantly impacts American families. Approximately one of every three adults in the United States will meet diagnostic criteria for a mental disorder sometime in his or her life, and 20% meet criteria for a mental disorder at any given time (Institute of Medicine 1994). The federal government estimates that between 4 and 5 million adults experience a serious mental illness (Barker et al. 1992); more than 3 million children and adolescents have serious emotional disorders that cause substantial functional impairment (Brandenburg et al. 1990). About 65 million youngsters, or 14%–20% of children from birth to age 18, have a diagnosable mental disorder (Brandenburg et al. 1990).

The costs of mental disorders and alcohol and drug abuse in the United States are enormous. Rice et al. (1991) estimated that the annual direct and indirect costs to society for mental health and substance abuse treatment exceeded $273 billion in 1988.

To meet unique and compelling needs of people with mental disorders, the public sector supports mental health service systems ranging from ambulatory mental health organizations and Veterans Administration medical centers to state and county mental hospitals. Each system provides a broad range of services within a continuum of care that targets the specific needs of certain populations.

In this chapter, we describe four unique service models that address the needs of people with mental disorders and how federal programs have advanced the cause of a continuum of care.

In recent years, there has been a dramatic shift in the way mental health services are financed and delivered. During the first half of this century, most people with long-term mental illness were housed in state or community mental hospitals. However, in the 1950s and 1960s, thousands of people who had been institutionalized were discharged from mental hospitals. Two factors contributed to this massive discharge. First, due to a series of breakthroughs in the psychopharmacology of mental illness and the availability of effective psychotropic medications, great numbers of patients could function outside hospital environments. Second, the general public became more accepting of the idea of providing mental health care to people within their communities rather than in faraway institutions. Thus, the community mental health movement was born.

Congress passed The Community Mental Health Centers Act in 1963. The act, based on the principle that persons with mental disabilities should be treated in the least restrictive environment possible, created a nationwide system of community mental health centers. The number of residents in public, state, and county mental hospitals fell rapidly, declining from about 559,000 in 1955 to 193,000 in 1975 to 72,000 in 1994 (Center for Mental Health Services 1995; Department of Health and Human Services 1981).

Most communities were ill prepared to meet the needs of deinstitutionalized individuals. At that time, the vast majority of community health centers did not offer the range of primary care, mental health, rehabilitation, and support services required by persons with long-term mental illness. As a result, many people with mental health disorders were unemployed and socially isolated, living in inadequate and substandard housing and lacking access to both physical and mental health care. Many ended up living on the streets—especially in the nation's urban centers—living proof that when deinstitutionalization occurred, communities often were not equipped to provide the comprehensive mental health and support services these individuals needed.

Community Support Systems for Adults With Long-Term, Disabling Mental Illness

Beginning in the late 1970s, the Public Health Service actively promoted the development of systems of care, commonly called "community support systems," for persons with long-term, disabling mental illness. To stimulate the development of community support systems, the Federal Community Support Program, which today is administered by the Center for Mental Health Services, has provided funds to all 50 states, the District of Columbia, and two territories (Stroul 1986). States and localities have created service programs with a simple philosophy in mind: developing innovative community support models that are organized, financed, and delivered in a way that is appropriate for the needs of the community.

Guiding Principles for Community Support Systems

Over time, the Public Health Service has issued a series of guiding principles intended to enhance the quality of service systems. These guiding principles advance the cause of the continuum of care by addressing the unique needs of individuals and the particular communities in which they live. Because the needs of individuals and the ability of communities to meet those needs are so varied, an ever-widening and responsive continuum of care is being created.

Guiding principles espoused by community support programs are reviewed below (Stroul 1984, 1988, 1989).

Personal dignity.   Services should be provided in an environment that protects privacy and enhances personal dignity.

Consumer centered.   Services should be based on the needs
of the patient.

Self-determination and empowerment.   Patients should retain the fullest possible control over their lives. As much as possible, patients should set personal goals and participate in
planning and evaluating public programs to reach these goals.

Culturally appropriate.   Services that are culturally appropriate should be available, accessible, and acceptable to everyone
needing them.

Flexibility.   Services should be available whenever necessary
and for as long as patients need support. They should be evaluated regularly and adapted to the unique and changing needs
and preferences of each patient.

Focus on strengths.   Services should build on the assets and
strengths of patients.

Normalization and incorporation of natural supports.
Services should be offered in the least restrictive and most natural settings possible. Patients should be encouraged to use common supports in the community and should be integrated into
the community's activities.

Special needs.   Services should be adapted to meet the needs
of specific subgroups of patients with serious mental illnesses, such
as individuals with both mental illness and substance abuse disorders or physical disabilities and people with mental illness who are
homeless or inappropriately placed within the correctional system.

Coordinated systems. The disparate components of the system must be brought together and made to work for the benefit of patients. At local, state, and national levels, collaboration requires formal cooperation among a broad range of public and private mental health and human service agencies.

Accountable systems. Service systems should be accountable to the users of the services and monitored by the state to ensure quality of care and relevance to the needs of patients. Patients and families should be involved in planning, implementing, monitoring, and evaluating services.

Clearly, the guiding principles reflect the ideal. Although states and communities may not be able to put all these ideas into practice immediately, they represent goals worth striving for.

Service System Components

The community support systems concept is not based on any one model for meeting the comprehensive needs of persons with chronic mental illness. Instead, it draws on elements of medical, rehabilitation, and social support models. Thus, each community should have service system components that perform the following functions (Stroul 1984, 1988, 1989).

Patient identification and outreach. Locate patients and reach out to inform them of available services. Ensure access to needed services and community resources by arranging for transportation, if necessary, or by taking the services to the patients. Help patients meet basic human needs for food, clothing, shelter, personal safety, and general medical and dental care. Assist them in applying for income, medical, housing, and other benefits that they may need and to which they are entitled.

Mental health treatment. Provide adequate mental health care, including diagnostic evaluation, supportive counseling,

psychotherapeutic treatment, and medication management services. Provide services to patients having both mental and substance abuse disorders.

Crisis response services.   Provide 24-hour, quick-response
crisis assistance that enables the patient, family, and friends to
cope with emergencies. Maintain the patient's status as a functioning community member to the greatest extent possible by
providing services such as a 24-hour hot line, walk-in crisis and
triage services, mobile outreach services for in-home crises, community crisis residential beds for temporary respite care, and
inpatient beds in a protective environment such as a psychiatric
unit of a general, community, or state hospital.

Health and dental care.   Provide accessible medical and dental services to people with serious mental illness who have significantly higher rates of physical illness than the general
population or who may have an undetected physical disease contributing to their mental disorder (Stroul 1989).

Housing.   Provide a range of rehabilitative and supportive
housing options for people not in crisis who need special living
arrangements with incentives and encouragement for self-
sufficiency.

Income supports and entitlements.   Help patients obtain
income supports and other entitlements needed for community
living by assisting with eligibility determination for public assistance or other programs, providing transportation to agencies,
and assisting with application forms.

Peer support.   Involve support systems, such as consumer
and family self-help groups and consumer-run service alternatives that provide social supports unavailable in formal systems
and can assist people who decline structured mental health services or who have moved beyond the need for them.

Family and community support.   Provide backup support, assistance, consultation, and education to families, friends, landlords, employers, community agencies, and others who come in frequent contact with patients to maximize benefits and minimize problems. Educate the public about mental illness to reduce stigma and promote community acceptance of people with mental disorders.

Rehabilitation services.   Provide a continuum of psychosocial services. Teach coping skills and daily and community living skills. Encourage the patient to develop outside interests and leisure time activities. Help patients find and use appropriate employment opportunities and vocational services.

Protection and advocacy.   Establish grievance procedures and mechanisms that conform with Public Law 99-319, The Protection and Advocacy for Individuals With Mental Illness Act of 1986. The act was designed to protect patient's rights both in and out of mental health or residential facilities.

Case management.   Facilitate patients' effective use of formal and informal helping systems, such as case management systems that designate a single person or team to help patients make informed choices about opportunities and services, ensure them timely access to needed assistance, provide opportunities and encouragement for self-help activities, and coordinate all services to meet patient goals.

Models of Community Support Services

The service needs of people with long-term mental disorders and the diverse resources of communities require a continuum of care. Many models of care have been developed with individual service philosophies and programmatic approaches (Liberman et al. 1984). Four models that have been implemented, tested, replicated, or adapted in a variety of environments are the 1) psychosocial rehabilitation model (Stroul 1986), 2) Fair-

weather Lodge model (Stroul 1986), 3) training in assertive
community treatment model (Drake and Burns 1995), and
4) consumer-run alternative model (Stroul 1986). The four models, supported in part by federal block grants to states, are briefly
described below.

Psychosocial rehabilitation model.   The psychosocial rehabilitation model (Stroul 1986) focuses on strengthening patients' skills and providing environmental supports necessary to
sustain them in the community. It also helps patients lead more
productive and satisfying lives. The model is usually organized
around a clubhouse or center. Patients, generally called members, are full participants in the operation of the program. The
model is nonmedical in that it emphasizes wellness rather than
illness, improving behavior rather than alleviating symptoms.

     With the center as the hub of activity, the model offers services that fall into five major areas: social/recreational, vocational,
residential, educational, and case management. *Social/recreational services* are designed to help members learn social and
interpersonal skills and to use leisure time constructively. They
foster a sense of community and healthy participation in normal
activities. *Vocational services* teach employment skills by providing practical work experience for members. *Residential services* provide shelter and a setting for practicing independent
living skills. *Educational services* develop basic academic skills,
as well as skills needed for community living. *Case management*
integrates all aspects of the model and helps members gain access to needed community resources such as mental health centers, welfare, social services, housing agencies, health and
recreation departments, the Social Security Administration, legal
aid, and so on.

     Psychosocial programs offer a range of other services. Some
programs have psychiatrists and nurses on staff to prescribe and
monitor medications. Others connect patients with outside
agencies for assistance with medications. Most services are provided indefinitely, functioning as continuous lifetime or periodic
supports for members who need them.

Data indicate that the psychosocial rehabilitation model is instrumental in decreasing the number of hospital admissions, shortening the length of hospital stays, and increasing employment rates (Stroul 1986). This model also is designed to improve academic and vocational performance (Cook and Solomon 1993), wages (Laird and Krown 1991), and residential independence (Cook et al. 1993).

The psychosocial rehabilitation model has been widely replicated. Fountain House, founded in New York City in 1948, was the first psychosocial rehabilitation center in the United States. In 1976, Fountain House received a federal grant to initiate a training program designed to help agencies establish services based on the psychosocial rehabilitation model.

Fairweather Lodge model. The Fairweather Lodge model (Stroul 1986) originated at a veterans' hospital in California in the 1960s. The model has two basic components: one in a hospital setting and the other in the community.

The hospital component is a transitional program designed to prepare patients for community living. In a small-group ward, 10–15 patients are taught skills in daily living, work, communication, and acceptable behavior and are encouraged to take increasing responsibility for their lives. Prepared members move to the community, where groups of 15–30 discharged patients live together in a homelike setting.

The community component is a lodge that provides a structured setting for day-to-day employment and peer support. It functions as a "business-commune," offering a supportive group living situation and responsible work. The lodge operates its own for-profit business, with patients as the workforce.

The Fairweather Lodge philosophy emphasizes that patients must have living skills, a job, and the support of family or friends to become contributing members of society and to cope with the stresses of everyday life. Its central premise is that the group exerts a powerful influence on members. The group establishes norms to follow and provides peer support. It creates an environment in which patients have status within their subcommunity and take mutual responsibility for each other's welfare. All activities are designed to enhance patients' collective control over their lives. In essence, the lodge is a small society that provides ex-hospital patients with the opportunity to be somewhat independent and have social acceptance and support.

Data indicate that recidivism rates and time spent in hospitals were lower and employment rates higher for Fairweather Lodge patients than they were for control subjects (Fairweather 1964; Fairweather et al. 1969) and that patients remain in the community longer than would be expected because of their history of hospitalizations (Fergus et al. 1990).

Sources of revenue for lodges include federal, state, and local mental health funds, as well as residents' Medicare, Medicaid, and Social Security monies. In addition, the federal government gave grants to the originators of the Fairweather Lodge to initiate dissemination efforts (Stroul 1986).

Training in assertive community treatment model. The premise of the training in assertive community treatment model (Drake and Burns 1995) is that both institutional and community programs fail to serve persons with the most severe impairments adequately. Its goals are to increase patients' length of time in the community, elevate their psychosocial functioning, minimize their psychiatric symptoms, and enhance their quality of life. It is grounded in the philosophy that managing the illness and providing support are more effective ways to maximize the functioning of people with severe mental disorders than attempting to cure the illness.

The training in assertive community treatment model also is built on the assumption that many problems leading to rehospitalizations are the result of poor coping skills. Thus, the model addresses four basic areas of life: daily living, vocational skills, leisure activities, and social/interpersonal relationships. The primary treatment intervention is teaching coping skills to the patient and his or her family and friends so they may be supportive of one another. Instead of preparing patients for community life, this model attempts to maintain patients in the community.

Clinical management, including monitoring symptoms and medications, is an integral part of the treatment. Patients are taught about their symptoms, the relationship of symptoms to environmental stresses, and the methods to control and manage symptoms.

Staff actively reach out to patients in their homes, workplaces, and other appropriate settings and are assertive in their approach. Home arrangements vary from independent living to more structured environments, such as halfway houses, foster homes, or board and care homes. Job situations range from full-time competitive employment to part-time sheltered work. Program services are normally available 24 hours a day and are of indefinite duration.

Data indicate that training in assertive community treatment improves clinical status, ability to work and live independently, social functioning, and compliance with medical instructions (Drake and Burns 1995). It is cost-effective (Drake and Burns 1995) and reduces hospitalizations (Dincin et al. 1993; Drake and Burns 1995).

Consumer-run alternative model.   In the consumer-run alternative model (Stroul 1986), current or former recipients of mental health services plan, administer, deliver, and evaluate mental health services. This model provides a peer support network that offers encouragement, support, assistance, and role models in a sensitive, nonjudgmental, and nonthreatening atmosphere.

This model is most often organized around a drop-in center. Anyone needing help can call or walk into the center to find acceptance, understanding, and a variety of structured and non-structured activities. Some meetings are for all members; others address specific problems such as finding a job, stopping smoking, and eating disorders. Peer counseling occurs informally in some centers and more formally in others. Some programs reach out to patients in hospitals, boarding homes, and other facilities.

Most consumer-run programs also provide social, recreational, and educational services. Many attempt to combat the stigma associated with mental illness through community education. Some provide advocacy and case management services. These programs help members access community resources such as housing, medical and legal services, and financial aid. At times, programs help patients avoid unwanted or unnecessary psychiatric interventions. Residential, crisis, and vocational services are provided less often.

Data suggest that this model has promise for many patients. Solomon and Draine (1995) found that over a 2-year period, a team of case managers who were also mental health consumers were as effective as a team of nonconsumer case managers in maintaining the stability of patients with severe mental disabilities.

People Who Are Homeless and Have a Mental Illness

To help people who are both homeless and have a mental illness, aid must encompass and integrate an enormous range of services and systems. Many systems that provide services to homeless individuals often do not work together. People with mental illness cannot readily negotiate and navigate a system in which health care, mental health and substance abuse treatment, social services, income support, legal services, housing, rehabilitation, and employment services are separate and uncoordinated. Leshner et al. (1992) laid out the essential elements of a system that can be accessible to and easily maneuvered by its intended users. Most of the elements were the same as those enumerated earlier in this chapter. However, the authors added other components.

The first such component is an assertive outreach program. Workers must meet and engage homeless people over long periods of time on their own terms and on their own turf.

The second is safe havens. People with mental illness who live on the streets need secure, clean, and stable housing where they can recuperate from the harsh street environment and develop necessary skills and linkages to benefits, treatment, and support. Unlike most shelters, these safe havens should place few demands on their guests. They should offer a place to stay during the day, the same bed each night, and secure storage areas for belongings.

Housing is essential, but it must be coordinated with services that can help people remain housed. A variety of housing options must be made affordable through a combination of approaches, including greater access to housing subsidies and increased employment opportunities.

At least half of those individuals who are both homeless and have a mental illness also suffer from alcohol or other drug abuse problems. People with co-occurring mental and substance use disorders require skilled assessment and access to detoxification, treatment, and recovery services specifically designed to deal with co-occurring problems.

An integrated system of care requires integrating basic life supports (e.g., food, clothing, and shelter) with specialized services (e.g., treatment). The federal government is promoting the integration of systems. For example, the Department of Health and Human Services, in collaboration with the Departments of Housing and Urban Development, Labor, Education, Veterans Affairs, and Agriculture, is making Access to Community Care and Effective Services and Supports (ACCESS) grants available to the states. This interdepartmental initiative is testing promising approaches to services integration in about 25 communities.

Other steps to promote systems integration include the development of two "memoranda of understanding" between the Department of Health and Human Services and other federal agencies. One with the Department of Justice is designed to find treatment settings for homeless people with severe mental illnesses who are placed inappropriately in jails. Another with the Departments of Labor and Education is designed to develop policies and programs that meet the rehabilitation and job training needs of homeless individuals who have a mental illness.

Systems of Care for Children and Adolescents With Serious Emotional Disturbances

Comprehensive community-based systems of care for children and adolescents with emotional disorders, and their families, in many ways mirrors those for adults. Systems of care for children and adolescents are based on the notion that services should be family focused and individualized, provided in the least restrictive and most clinically appropriate treatment environment, coordinated among multiple agencies, and culturally sensitive (Stroul 1993).

The federal government, through a series of Child and Adolescent Service System Program (CASSP) demonstration grants and other agency initiatives, has supported the development of accessible and appropriate service delivery systems for children and adolescents with serious emotional disorders and their families. These grants help states to create comprehensive, coordinated systems of care for children.

Guiding Principles for Systems of Care for Children and Adolescents

Some systems needs for children and adolescents are different from those for adults. The rapidly changing mental and physical status of children and adolescents requires more frequent reassessments of clinical interventions. Children's dependence on adult caregivers requires the caregivers to be actively and continually engaged in planning and care. The frequent entry of children into mental health systems of care through schools, juvenile justice, and child welfare agencies requires these agencies to function as integrated wholes. Finally, account should be taken of the differences in legal status between children and adults.

CASSP conceptualized a philosophy and system of care for children and adolescents with emotional disorders. Guiding principles that supplement those for adults are as follows (Stroul and Friedman 1986, 1996).

Comprehensive array of services. Children with emotional disturbances should have access to a comprehensive array of services that address their physical, emotional, social, and educational needs.

Individualized service plans. Services tailored to the unique needs and potentials of each child should be rendered and guided by an individualized service plan.

Family involvement. Families and surrogate families should be full participants in all aspects of the planning and delivery of services.

Early intervention. Early identification and intervention should be promoted to enhance the likelihood of positive outcomes.

Transition to adult services. Smooth transitions to the adult service system should be ensured as children with emotional disturbances reach maturity.

Protection of rights. The rights of children with emotional disturbances should be protected, and effective advocacy for them should be promoted.

Service System Components

A system of care for children with serious emotional disturbances is a continuum of mental health and other necessary services designed to meet multiple and changing needs (Stroul and Friedman 1986, 1996). One good model for a system of care that can be used as a guide in planning and policymaking has eight major dimensions of service: mental health, social, education, physical health, substance abuse, vocational, recreation, and operational services.

Operational components include case management, juvenile justice, family support, advocacy, transportation, and "wraparound" and other services (Stroul and Friedman 1986, 1996).

In most community care sites, diagnoses in the disruptive disorders category, such as attention-deficit/hyperactivity disorder and conduct disorder, are most common. A majority of the children served under these community systems are boys who are behind educationally and have a history of psychiatric hospitalization (Stroul 1993). Many have exhibited behaviors considered dangerous to themselves or others. In addition, many live in poverty in single-parent households and have been abused physically and sexually. Many families also have histories of mental illness and chemical dependence (Stroul 1993).

Depending on needs, communities offer a continuum of services in nonresidential and residential settings. Nonresidential services include outpatient services for individuals and for families and groups, home-based services, day treatment, crisis services, after-school and evening programs, therapeutic respite services, behavioral aide services, and parent education and support. Residential services include therapeutic foster care, therapeutic group care, crisis residential services, residential treatment services, and inpatient hospital services.

There are differences between the systems of care developed by these communities and traditional service systems for children with emotional disorders. Some of the differences are outlined as follows:

- *Expanded "intermediate" services.* Intensive treatment services in more normalized environments can often be used as alternatives to hospitalization. Home-based services, day treatment, and therapeutic foster care are examples of community continuum of care services.
- *Individualized services.* Care is adapted to the needs of each child and family.
- *Multidisciplinary and interagency teams.* Representatives of agencies involved with each child and family function as a treatment and services planning team.

- *Case management.* Conceptually, case managers for children provide services similar to those for adults. They are the ultimate monitor of the patient and coordinator of all the services that the patient needs.

There is evidence that the care provided for children with serious emotional disturbances in community-based facilities reduces the number of admissions to hospitals, residential treatment centers, and juvenile detention centers. It also appears to improve functioning, mood, and interpersonal relationships, as well as to decrease alcohol and drug use and other undesirable behaviors (Stroul 1993).

Discussion

Although new, innovative community mental health services continue to be created, not everyone embraces their implementation or underlying tenets. Some decry an overemphasis on social reform rather than clinical treatment; others argue that the community mental health centers encourage demedicalization and deprofessionalization (Thompson 1994).

The dominant trend since the early 1980s has been the curtailment of services. Efforts to reduce health care costs, coupled with the belief by many that mental disorders are moral problems rather than illnesses, help to drive this trend (Thompson 1994).

States and localities have traditionally been responsible for the care of people with serious mental illness, but distinctions between public and private care have blurred. Rather than provide services directly, states increasingly purchase, regulate, and monitor services provided by private and nonprofit institutions in managed care environments (Mechanic 1994).

To avoid unanticipated consequences during the rush to managed care, it may be useful to examine some similarities between deinstitutionalization and current managed care activities. Kane (1995) delineated their similar goals and problems. She pointed out that managed care plans purport to promote comprehensive health care services at reduced costs. These goals are similar to those promoted in the 1960s as outcomes of community mental health care centers. She also marked commonalities in their lack of agreement about the meaning of basic terms, the rapid downsizing of medical centers and hospitals, and the lack of comprehensive planning or evaluation to ensure appropriate outpatient delivery services with qualified staff.

Legislative mandates and a plethora of constituencies make it difficult for government bureaucracies to be as flexible as private institutions. Nevertheless, the public sector is obliged to continually require, monitor, and assess the development of workable solutions for old and new problems. Practitioners should be trained to collaborate in interdisciplinary teams. Safeguards should be developed to prevent the arrogation of mental health resources to medical care. Effectiveness of services for people with severe and persistent mental illness should be judged by patients' functional levels, rates of deterioration, and quality of life rather than by cures.

Professional, consumer, family, and advocacy groups must be constantly vigilant. They also must work with governments at all levels to recognize problems rapidly and make concerted efforts to solve them quickly.

Conclusion

A flexible, broad continuum of care must be supported for people with mental illnesses whose needs vary greatly. Although everyone requires certain basic commodities, such as food, clothing, and shelter, these can be provided in many different ways. There is no universally accepted way to provide the necessities of life and other vital services. Each child and adult with a severe emotional or mental disorder is a unique individual with combinations of needs unlike those of anyone else. Delivery of services should be tailored to the needs of the individuals requiring care.

Appropriate, timely mental health services reduce society's economic, social, and personal burdens. As public and private institutions are looking for ways to limit resources for health care, there is an increasing recognition of the interrelatedness of mental and physical health. People with severe mental illness tend to ignore or mistreat their physical selves, and thus increase costs for their medical treatments. Proper attention to the mental state of people with serious physical ailments can mitigate medical symptoms and prolong life. Mental illness and its consequences for families and children who are vulnerable spill over to communities and neighborhoods.

Mental health care systems are changing rapidly. Limited resources make it necessary for services to be provided as cost-effectively as possible, and services provided in the community are generally less expensive than those provided in hospitals. Productively employed people benefit society even if employment entails a large measure of support. Therefore, the federal government has supported, and will continue to support, a broad array of services that advance the idea and the reality of a continuum of care.

References

Barker PR, Manderscheid RW, Hendershot GE, et al: Serious mental illness and disability in the adult household population: United States, 1989, in Center for Mental Health Services and National Institute of Mental Health: Mental Health, United States, 1992 (DHHS Publ No SMA-92-1942). Edited by Manderscheid RW, Sonnenschein MA. Washington, DC, U.S. Government Printing Office, 1992, pp 255–261

Brandenburg N, Friedman R, Silver S: The epidemiology of childhood psychiatric disorders: prevalence findings from recent studies. J Am Acad Child Adolesc Psychiatry 29:76–83, 1990

Center for Mental Health Services: Additions and Resident Patients at End of Year, State and County Mental Hospitals, by Age and Diagnosis, by State, United States, 1994. Rockville, MD, Center for Mental Health Services, 1995

Cook JA, Solomon ML: The community scholar program: an outcome study of supported education for students with severe mental illness. Psychosocial Rehabilitation Journal 17:83–97, 1993

Cook JA, Kozlowski-Graham K, Razzanol L: Psychosocial rehabilitation of deaf persons with severe mental illness: a multivariate model of residential outcomes. Rehabilitation Psychology 38:261–274, 1993

Department of Health and Human Services: Toward a national plan for the chronically mentally ill: report to the Secretary by the Department of Health and Human Services Steering Committee on the Chronically Mentally Ill (DHHS Publ No ADM-81-1077). Washington, DC, Department of Health and Human Services, 1981

Dincin J, Wasmer D, Witheridge TF, et al: Impact of assertive community treatment on the use of state hospital inpatient bed-days. Hospital and Community Psychiatry 44:833–838, 1993

Drake RE, Burns BJ: Special section on assertive community treatment: an introduction. Psychiatr Serv 46:667–668, 1995

Fairweather GW (ed): Social Psychology in Treating Mental Illness: An Experimental Approach. New York, Wiley, 1964

Fairweather GW, Sanders D, Cressler D, et al: Community Life for the Mentally Ill: An Alternative to Hospitalization. Chicago, IL, Aldine, 1969

Fergus EO, Bryant BD, Balzell AI: The lodge society in Michigan: a follow-up study. Paper presented at the annual meeting of the American Psychiatric Association, New York, April 1990

Institute of Medicine: Reducing Risks for Mental Disorders. Washington, DC, National Academy Press, 1994

Kane CF: Deinstitutionalization and managed care: deja vu?, Nursing Update 46:883–884, 889, 1995

Laird M, Krown S: Evaluation of a transitional employment program. Psychosocial Rehabilitation Journal 15:3–8, 1991

Leshner AI, Britten G, Carlile P, et al: Outcasts on Main Street: report of the Federal Task Force on Homelessness and Severe Mental Illness, Interagency Council on the Homeless (DHHS Publ No ADM-92-1904). Washington, DC, Department of Health and Human Services, 1992

Liberman R, Kuehnel T, Phipps C, et al: Resource Book for Psychiatric Rehabilitation: Elements of Service for the Mentally Ill. Camarill, CA, Center for Rehabilitation Research and Training in Mental Illness, UCLA School of Medicine, 1984

Mechanic D: Integrating mental health into a general health care system. Hospital and Community Psychiatry 45:893–897, 1994

Rice DP, Kelman S, Miller LS: Estimates of economic costs of alcohol and drug abuse and mental illness, 1985 and 1988. Public Health Rep 106:280–292, 1991

Solomon P, Draine J: The efficacy of a consumer case management team: 2-year outcomes of a randomized trial. Journal of Mental Health Administration 22:135–146, 1995

Stroul BA: Toward Community Support Systems for the Mentally Disabled: the NIMH Community Support Program. Boston, MA, Boston University Center for Rehabilitation Research and Training in Mental Health, 1984

Stroul BA: Models of Community Support Services: Approaches to Helping Persons With Long-Term Mental Illness. Boston, MA, Center for Psychiatric Rehabilitation, 1986

Stroul BA: Community Support Systems for Persons With Long-Term Mental Illness: Questions and Answers. Rockville, MD, National Institute of Mental Health Community Support Program, 1988

Stroul BA: Community support systems for persons with long-term mental illness: a conceptual framework. Psychosocial Rehabilitation Journal 12:9–26, 1989

Stroul BA: Systems of Care for Children and Adolescents With Severe Emotional Disturbances: What Are the Results? Washington, DC, Georgetown University Child Development Center, Child and Adolescent Service System Program Technical Assistance Center, 1993

Stroul BA, Friedman RM: A System of Care for Children and Adolescents With Severe Emotional Disturbances. Washington, DC, Georgetown University Child Development Center, National Technical Assistance Center for Children's Mental Health, 1986

Stroul BA, Friedman RM: The system of care concept and philosophy, in Children's Mental Health: Creating Systems of Care in a Changing Society. Edited by Stroul BA. Baltimore, MD, Paul H Brookes, 1996, pp 3–21

Thompson JW: Trends in the development of psychiatric services, 1844–1994. Hospital and Community Psychiatry 45:987–992, 1994

21

Beyond the Continuum: Community, Family, and Consumer Services

Laurie M. Flynn

At age 17, Shannon seemed to have everything going for her. A high school senior, she was at the top of her class. Her academic talents were matched by other abilities. Shannon starred in her high school musical, was a prize-winning poet, and was a gifted amateur painter. She also was active in her community, singing in a church choir and tutoring a foreign student learning English as a second language.

Early in her senior year, however, Shannon became ill with what was later diagnosed as a severe depressive illness. Her family hospitalized her just before Thanksgiving, when Shannon was in a catatonic and suicidal state. Because of continuing discrimination in health care coverage, precisely 30 days after admittance Shannon was discharged to her family. Fragile, just beginning to respond to antidepressants, Shannon came home. Her psychiatrist indicated that she should not return to school, at least for awhile. The hospital indicated she should continue outpatient psychiatric services and gave the family the address of a community mental health center.

In the early weeks following discharge, Shannon's family discovered that the medically based continuum of services is incomplete and inadequate. As they later reported, "we simply had to invent a program because, astonishingly enough, there was none."

Too frail to return to school, Shannon still needed something to do with her time and energy. Her family pieced together their own effort at rehabilitation. Because the parents were able to coordinate their work schedules, Shannon spent part of each day with one of her parents. As she gained strength and became more interested in outside activities, Shannon spent part of each day in one of their work settings as a volunteer support person. Later, with the encouragement of her family, Shannon sought and found a part-time job at a day care center. Throughout the spring, as she recovered more of her self-esteem, she increased her hours at the day care center. She also began gradually to return to the activities that had formerly given her life meaning and focus.

All of these activities—doing volunteer work, working part-time jobs, returning to art classes and choir, and becoming involved in a support group for individuals with depressive disorders—were arranged by Shannon's family or by Shannon herself. All of these nonmedical, informal parts of the continuum of care are viewed by Shannon and her family, 10 years later, as crucial elements in her recovery.

It has been widely recognized for a decade or more that our traditional mental health system, both public and private, is not truly a system at all. Rather, it is a patchwork of unconnected services of varying qualities. One critic has charged that our mental health service system is more thought disordered than many of the people it is trying to serve. This well-documented fragmentation of services leads to difficulty in accessing them for many patients. Poor coordination between services and service providers often discourages patients, who soon give up attempting to put back together the pieces of their lives. This is especially true when traditional medical and mental health services are not allied with other life needs, such as housing, rehabilitation, and vocational training and employment.

The role that stigma plays in undermining coordination of services is also important. Simply stated, many patients do not like and do not want to associate themselves with most traditional mental health programs. A number of studies have shown that for individuals most in need of such community-based services (those with severe mental illnesses), less than three-fourths are still connected to the formal service system 6 months after discharge from inpatient care. Surveys of patients indicate that the stigmatizing element, the often infantile and demeaning focus of many day treatment programs, and the lack of attention directed toward getting on with life are all reasons for dropping out. In an era when mainstreaming has been so important in the disability movement broadly, our community mental health programs still lag far behind.

Patients want activities directed toward recovery. They want to do things that are age appropriate and that lead to less dependence on medical and mental health services. Yet too many of our mental health centers and other outpatient programs rely on traditional therapy groups, activity groups, recreation groups, and specialized and artificially developed programs that often feature activities such as making macramé plant holders and weaving doormats. As one patient said to me, "There's certainly a lot of subliminal messages when a 35-year-old person in good physical and mental shape is asked to spend the afternoons making doormats out of straw."

As managed care takes hold in medical and health delivery systems, we need to pay close attention to what patients and their families tell us about the kind of support they need once daily medical attention is no longer required. As Shannon's family discovered, the mental health community must, in fact, reinvent aftercare that it may not directly control and that may look very different from what has been previously seen as part of the continuum. Such supports must be based on several important principles:

- Children, adolescents, and adults need a wider range of choices as they move from intensive inpatient treatment settings to outpatient and community-centered services. "One size does *not* fit all" is a truism that we must remember as we tailor mental health services in the future.

- Because of stigma and because of the lack of relevance of many of the older service models, we must move rapidly toward normalization and mainstreaming both the location and the focus of community care. The recovery model of mental illness, even for those with severe disorders, is an important foundation for new thinking. Patients and their families need to and must become independent more rapidly. Not only must they be put in charge of their own illnesses, but they also must be given increasing responsibility for life management. In this paradigm, the diagnosis of a mental disorder is not a sentence to a lifetime of illness, dependency, and isolation.

- In the future, the continuum of care must be consumer centered, family respectful, individually tailored, mainstreamed, and outcome driven. Many of the services and supports will not be provided by professionals.

What are the elements that extend beyond the traditional continuum of care as defined in psychiatric services? Each of these core parts of the fabric of recovery is interwoven with appropriate psychiatric care and rehabilitation programs.

Family

Families of individuals with mental illnesses have too often been blamed as the cause of the illness or discounted as key elements in the continuum of care. Yet statistics tell us that 65% of individuals who are discharged from psychiatric hospitals return to their family homes. All too often, these families are poorly prepared to play the critical role they have been given. Educated, informed, and supported families are a vital part of the informal system of care that will be increasingly viable in the future. The National Alliance for the Mentally Ill (NAMI) has been in the forefront of helping families succeed in this role. Through more than 1,000 support groups and chapters in all 50 states, families everywhere can find in each other the information and coping skills that are necessary as they provide day-to-day encouragement to their recovering relative. Through family-to-family education programs, such as the Journey of Hope, those families who have years of experience with loved ones who have a mental illness are able to teach and assist families newly involved with psychiatric services. Because our mental health system, both public and private, is unable to meet the needs of all individuals who seek help, support for the vital role of families as partners in care must be central to developing mental health policy in the future. Outmoded confidentiality policies, which prohibit family caregivers from understanding even the basic requirements of their role, must be challenged.

Consumer Self-Help Groups

More individuals with mental illnesses are finding that they can help one another, just as organizations such as NAMI have served their families well through support, education, and advocacy. Over the past decade, the mental health consumers movement has grown rapidly. The elements that patients value most include the opportunities to meet, talk, and make friends with others who have experienced a psychiatric disorder, as well as the opportunity to share practical and daily coping skills. Mental illness is a uniquely isolating disease. The stigma still unfairly attached to psychiatric disorders isolates individuals who need friends and companions as they work to rebuild their identity and self-esteem after a major psychiatric episode. Compassion, understanding, good humor, and patience are all important parts of such a circle of friendship. Self-help groups, including the National Depressive and Manic Depressive Association, the National Mental Health Consumers Association, Recovery Incorporated, Schizophrenics Anonymous, and others are playing an important role in supplementing the medical care that is the cornerstone of recovery from mental illness. Friendships forged in these sharing and caring settings enable people to withstand the inevitable stresses, crises, and difficulties that face all of us and that are so threatening to people with a serious mental illness. Some patients have even started their own programs, including "drop-in centers" and patient-run services. Often undervalued, family and patient self-help groups are indeed important predictors of compliance with treatment, reduction in inpatient days, and ultimate recovery of function and prevention of disability. Managed care executives and others designing reimbursement policies in the health care system of the future would do well to create incentives for caregiving families and patients to participate in the important work and support provided by self-help groups.

Church and Community

Serious mental illness has a profound impact on each individual it touches, shaking the core of self-confidence and often upsetting the life plans so carefully made. Mental illness too often robs patients of their future. Community groups and churches can play an important role in helping individuals with psychiatric illnesses to reintegrate into the mainstream. Spiritual dimensions, frequently commented on by those in psychiatry, and the historic role of conscience that the church and religious community have played are evident in the network of day programs, outreach services, crisis centers, and shelters provided by churches and synagogues throughout the country. Another aspect of this work, however, often goes unmentioned. Patients and their families find that volunteering in these settings and participating in religious life is a beginning of the hope that leads to change. The religious community, with its traditional emphasis on helping those with disabilities and promoting tolerance and acceptance, can be an important touchstone for renewing self-confidence as patients are discharged earlier from inpatient care. Civic organizations, such as the Kiwanis, Rotary, Lions Club, and others, offer the same opportunities to many patients and provide educational and support programs in hundreds of cities and towns across the nation. As the stigma of mental illness slowly recedes, these activities in thousands of communities will ultimately mainstream individuals with mental illness.

Recreation, Hobbies, and Personal Interests

For many patients, a major psychiatric break marks the end of their dreams. Many former patients comment bitterly that after their psychiatric disorder was diagnosed, it became their only known identity. Because mental illness can affect so many areas of life and because services have been both difficult to access and hard to sustain, mentally ill individuals find themselves cut off from the activities that build color and interest in the lives of others. Recreation, hobbies, and personal interests are an important part of the continuum that extends well beyond the medical model. Paying attention to their physical health, individuals with mental illnesses are building strength that indeed may translate into improved mental health. We know that psychiatric illness is a predictor of early death and that individuals with mental illnesses often have undiagnosed and untreated physical illnesses as well. Exercising regularly, participating in sports, and joining a gym or a community team are not just interesting ways to spend time, but such activities can be a vital part of the continuum of care. Similarly, as patients work to re-

build their self-esteem, parts of their lives that have been important to them must be rebuilt. Whether the former interest was
in sailing or singing, art or athletics, these definers of individu-
ality are crucial to recovery. Too often, they are not viewed as an
important component of community services and rehabilitation.

Education and Employment

Many individuals with mental illnesses are first affected while
they are still pursuing their education. Psychiatric hospitalization interrupts or ends this education for too many people.
The challenge of education, the inherent normalization it offers,
and the important new identity as "student" that it provides all
make school an important part of the informal system of care.
William Anthony and his colleagues at the Boston University Research and Training Center have demonstrated how important
and how successful supported education can be for mentally ill
individuals. The Americans With Disabilities Act provides us with
the next level of challenge. As more patients recover from many
of their symptoms, they are looking for the opportunity to work.
Indeed, many have observed that work is good therapy. It provides many of the key elements to recovery. It is an automatic
social milieu where individuals may make friendships easily
around shared tasks. It provides a regular structure and offers
some continuity and meaning from day to day. Work, especially
when it is paid, offers some independence to the too many mentally ill individuals who live on the margins of poverty. Yet, public
policy continues to discourage this ultimate step in the recovery
process. Patients who are able to work full-time frequently find
they jeopardize their access to Medicaid, which is a poverty-
based program. "If you recover too much and really get well,"
said one patient, "the first thing that happens is you lose the only
medical care you can get." Because of all of these problems, it is
clear that in the future the continuum of care for mentally ill
persons must include a far greater focus on continuing educa-

tion, training, and opportunities for meaningful, paid employment.

All of these elements of the continuum of care extend well beyond the traditional service paradigm. What is striking about these new sources of help—family and friends, church and community, self-help groups, recreation, hobbies, personal interests, education, and employment—is that none of them is a part of traditional mental health service programming. As we look to the use of resources in the future, it is important to remind ourselves continually that not everything we need or want for patients can or should come out of the "mental health box." Given what we know about the pernicious impact of stigma and the clear patterns of refusal and denial of service needs that are associated with stigma, patients are pointing the way to a new paradigm. Medical crisis and community care must of course be grounded in psychiatric and mental health providers. But much of what makes for the fabric of life is best accepted and most useful when it is provided through the regular community channels.

A service provider in a poor southern state demonstrated the integration of mental health and community services extremely well. Because the mental health budget was small, this provider, a social worker, had only a converted warehouse as her mental health rehabilitation center. Because her budget was small, she quickly realized she could provide only a basic meeting ground or clubhouse-type program in the converted warehouse. Yet, she knew how boring and isolating such group therapy sessions can become. She had several hundred patients referred, and she did not want to lose any, so early in the program she surveyed patients about their interests and dreams. What had they been involved in before their illness struck? What talents did they have? What interests and hopes did they have for their future? She specifically asked what strengths they thought they could offer.

Thus, the program was built. Then, the social worker turned away from the mental health community and looked toward the larger community where other citizens contribute and draw resources. She went to the garden club and asked if they might accept two or three people who indicated an interest and a green thumb. She did not start a horticulture program separate from the community. Instead, she integrated and mainstreamed those at the clubhouse who were interested in flowers. She went to the community little theater and placed five or six others in that activity. Again, she did not start a special theater troupe for mentally ill persons. She took mentally ill persons to the existing theater troupe and helped make a place for them. Similarly, she got people involved in Little League baseball as umpires and ticket takers. Some participated at the local YMCA as swimming coaches and in aerobics classes. A local retirement center took several individuals as part-time aides to the elderly, and the local junior high was happy to have some help in its carpentry classes.

In all of these cases, two things were evident. Most of the continuum of community care is now available but simply closed to mentally ill persons. By taking into consideration the strengths and stated needs of individuals with mental illnesses, we can motivate and truly support their individual identities. The mental health box does not need to become bigger and more comprehensive to serve those who have mental illnesses. It may need to become smaller, more focused, and more specialized, and mental health professionals may need to see themselves as "brokers" in mainstreaming patients. This specialization is what patients and families would consider success. Individuals with arthritis, diabetes, or a heart condition can and do fully participate in as much of the community's life as they are able to and interested in. Mentally ill persons can and should, too. The separation, isolation, and unimaginative programming that have characterized community care for the past 20 years must change. The mental health consumer movement for patients and families—built on self-help, belief in recovery, and insistence on an end to discrimination—has laid the groundwork for a continuum of care that is truly comprehensive, fully integrated, and more acceptable to patients and their families.

V

Conclusion

22 Learning to Manage Care

Robert K. Schreter, M.D.

Steven S. Sharfstein, M.D., M.P.A.

Carol A. Schreter, M.S.W., Ph.D.

Managed care, driven by economics, has caused a revolution in psychiatry. There used to be just two major treatment options. Outpatient care, the 50-minute hour, most often involved weekly sessions and was partly paid out of pocket by the patient. Inpatient psychiatric care, covered by insurance, started with a 30-day evaluation and often extended into many months. Other options, including medical and nonmedical supports, were developed in the 1960s and 1970s by the public sector. These options, however, have been largely ignored by private insurers.

Advances in psychopharmacology and psychosocial treatments now allow patients to be treated outside of the hospital. Instead of being hospitalized for 3 months, a patient may stay in the hospital for just 3–5 days and then move to a day treatment program and halfway house for several days, weeks, or months. Intensity of care and location have been uncoupled. The hospital is no longer seen as the first place for treatment but as a last resort when alternatives fail. For the first time, money is available for other options.

A guiding principle of managed care, dictated by third-party payers, is the principle of parsimony. Clinicians are expected to provide the least intensive, least expensive treatment option, unless another can be proven more effective. This is an era of experimentation and healthy competition, when payers are beginning to "let all flowers bloom." Programs developing over the past 20 years are being refined and replicated. Most controversial, however, is that the goals of treatment are also being dictated by payers. Payers expect patients to stabilize and return to function better, not to be cured.

In this context, clinicians struggle to make the necessary choices when recommending a mode of treatment for a particular patient. This volume is an early effort to describe the developing programs and treatment options. For mental health care, this is a how-to book. Clinical innovators describe existing best efforts so that readers can learn how to set up and use the emerging "continuum of care."

The Continuum Is Flexible

In Sections I and II, enthusiastic clinical innovators describe individual components of this emerging continuum. They clearly define whom they can and cannot treat. There are many recurring themes. It seems that most segments start with a particular patient population and then expand in both directions, serving people with greater or lesser or different needs. The reader may sense considerable overlap. All along the continuum, programs seem to be treating people in crisis. Only for one population, people seen as clearly dangerous to themselves or others, is there an automatic indication for only one level of care. In the interest of safety, these patients require acute hospital admission. For most other patients, it is not yet possible to say with certainty who is best treated where. Levels of care, and their boundaries, are not yet as clearly distinguished from one an-other as they probably will be in the future. Medical necessity criteria and indications for admission are not yet well defined.

High-functioning patients now get short-term, episodic, out-patient treatment. Others, it seems, may go to any of several players along the continuum. Perhaps assigning patients to pro-grams is like dealing a deck of cards. Does assignment to a pro-gram then matter? At this point, perhaps similar patients do not need the same program but the same opportunity for effective treatment.

The more disturbed patients may experience the continuum as a linear sequence, with programs more or less structured, more or less intensive. These patients tend to move from higher to lower levels of care as their conditions respond to treatment. Healthier patients are more likely to see the continuum as a set of choices from which they or their providers can select a treat-ment option.

In Section II, "Using the Continuum for Children, Adoles-cents, and the Elderly," psychiatric subspecialists describe how the continuum can be adapted to different age groups. The el-derly with cognitive decline need mental health services at nursing homes or life-care communities. Children may need su-pervised housing for just 2 or 3 days, a cooling-off place, while clinicians work with the family. It seems that continuum compo-nents are multiplying. Housing may involve a housing contin-uum—programs with different purposes, different expectations regarding length of stay and function, different levels of treat-ment and supervision.

In terms of program structure, each level of care already has some unique characteristics, including differences in

- Location (at hospital, in community, or freestanding)
- Physical plant
- Size of patient population
- Hours of service per day
- Staffing (composition, ratio, medical versus nonmedical)
- Types/intensity of services offered

- Family involvement
- Goals
- Anticipated length of stay
- Cost

The continuum can be an internal network within a base institution. Insurers and providers are establishing giant, vertically integrated systems of care. Or, it can be a network of more loosely associated providers and community supports. A continuum can be set up within a single facility. For instance, an inpatient unit may also welcome outpatients, providing partial hospital care. A patient may at first attend 7 days a week for intensive treatment and then come less often, phased down to 2 days a week for supportive rehabilitation, at the same site. Another example follows.

> Over the past 7 years, Ms. S was admitted to the psychiatric hospital almost annually for periods of 60–90 days. Last year, under managed care, she was admitted to the hospital for 10 days for crisis intervention and then spent 2 weeks in partial hospital care during the day and a supervised living arrangement at night. On discharge from the partial hospital, she spent another 14 days sleeping at the supervised shelter.
>
> Because Ms. S had a recurring condition requiring costly care, she was followed by a case manager. They spoke monthly by telephone or as needed. Ms. S and her therapist maintained contact on a more frequent basis. The therapist was also in contact with the case manager. This year, when the case manager sensed that Ms. S was beginning to relapse, Ms. S was moved quickly into the partial hospital. In this way, Ms. S avoided acute 24-hour inpatient care this year.

In Sections I and II, the authors seem to be saying that less costly continuum options work for many patients. A social worker and nurse making an initial assessment by home visit can cost $400, as opposed to $800 for the first day's assessment in an institution. This assessment can even be done in a shelter for the homeless. Subsequent home visits may cost $175, as opposed to $600 per day in a psychiatric hospital.

Early studies predicted that drastically shorter hospital stays would lead to catastrophe, such as recently discharged patients committing suicide. Now, when a 14-year-old boy, for example, is acutely depressed, he may be hospitalized for just 4 days. In such a brief evaluation, the treatment team may fail to recognize that the focus of treatment should be the mother. But time has shown that such obvious failures are much less common than expected. Many patients seem to benefit from resolving their problems while living outside, in the community.

With such a continuum, patients develop alliances with a "hub" program rather than an alliance with a therapist. Patients may like having options and greater freedom. High-functioning patients may never see the continuum as more than a matter of choice, of options. Chronic care patients may move from one layer of care to another, receiving intensive care from different programs over time. The continuum is then a "hospital without walls." With the patient in mind, programs are becoming more accessible by location, by having evening hours, and by providing telephone consultations.

In a system with multiple layers and providers, the best clinicians may be those who have the best Rolodex (i.e., the best referral system) and good relations with other treatment facilities. Psychiatrists will be most valued for their special skills in evaluation, diagnosis, and treatment planning. They will be asked to

- Review all patients for possible medications.
- Provide emergency management for the most difficult, most unstable, or deteriorating patients.
- Advise lesser-trained team members with their most difficult patients.

The psychiatrist also should be involved in the gatekeeping process (assigning new patients to programs), should back up the person who answers the telephone, and should be available, when necessary, to see new patients face-to-face. Errors at the outset can put patients and families at risk of grave harm. But the role of the psychiatrist is not yet determined at lower levels of care. Housing options tend to be run by social workers. Drop-in centers may be run by ex-patients. In using the clinical Rolodex, psychiatrists must learn to function as team members. They may not always lead this team.

Management Is Costly

If the continuum is a response to cost controls, driven by economics, is it cost-effective? Section III, "Planning and Administering the Continuum," deals first with this critical issue. Cost controls seem to depend on how well the components are integrated by teamwork, case management, and automated flow of information. Moving the most ill patients up and down the continuum requires interaction between programs and professions, an ever-widening treatment team. Information must flow with the patient. Many people involved at different layers can result in wasted time in meetings and duplicate assessments and reports. Should a patient's chart and laboratory tests move from one provider to another? Is the concept of patient confidentiality to be abandoned? When payers switch managed care companies from year to year, a new set of providers is introduced. This, too, is wasteful. We do not yet know how to follow a single patient through multiple levels of the continuum.

Administration is costing 5%–30% of the total mental health care bill. This shifts money from the clinical to the administrative side. Managed care generates greatest savings early in the process as physicians change their behavior—where inpatient stays are shortened or avoided entirely. But after that, the "managing" process may simply add to total costs.

Section III also describes current attempts to automate the mental health delivery process. This allows for accountability and the possibility of measuring patient outcomes. Computers can help clinicians decide where a particular patient should be treated by suggesting several treatment choices.

Throughout this volume, one reads about the need for published admission criteria, treatment guidelines, and outcome studies. Although the computerized tracking of patients can help, is it possible to standardize a moving target?

Clearly, the continuum concept produces some major problems, including

- Making placement decisions with no criteria guide
- Moving patients quickly between programs to lower levels of care
- Providing continuity of care when people move in the continuum between programs
- Getting crucial clinical information to flow between programs
- Developing treatment guidelines describing physical plant, service components, or staffing patterns for the various treatment options

Despite these serious problems, Sharfstein and Kent (Chapter 18, in this volume) provide a case example of the transformation of a mental hospital to a health system. Why does the hospital go through this painful restructuring process? From the ethical view, this is necessary when a third-party payer will not authorize hospitalization. From the pragmatic view, a hospital transforms itself to survive and continue its mission. The inpatient unit functions more flexibly, serving more people for shorter stays as well as others for outpatient, day treatment, and partial hospital care.

Lessons From the Public Sector

In the public sector since the 1960s, funds were always capped, and community mental health centers also found the need to

expand services. They ultimately moved to providing nonmedical supports—supported housing, jobs, and social programs.
These are not yet covered by private insurers. New housing programs also face regulatory constraints from the medical accreditation organizations or from the local or state medical or housing
authorities.

Section IV, "Public Policy Issues and the Continuum," begins
to reveal the holes in the continuum. When the most costly patients use up private insurance, they tend to be "dumped" into
public sector care. This is not a smooth transition between systems. Speaking for families, the National Alliance for the Mentally Ill says *continuum* is a misnomer. What actually occurs is
increased fragmentation of services. Families are not prepared
for time-limited, daytime-only services, where people are sent
home quicker and sicker. Families are at a disadvantage because
patient information is treated as confidential and not shared
with the family. The family says, "How can you send this person
home so soon? We are not ready. He threatened to kill me just 3
days ago." Apparently the tension between families and providers is increasing, even when patients benefit from outpatient
treatment options.

If expanding the continuum by adding nonmedical supports
is critical, as the families and the public sector experience suggest, will it be necessary for the public sector to force a broader
view of mental health care onto the private care continuum?

Do Patients Benefit?

In all, this volume is a first effort at learning how to manage care,
not just dollars. It shows the current developments and limitations in our ability to manage care. It describes the struggle to
find answers. It will be important to take what we have learned
from the public sector, from the community mental health center experience, and apply it on behalf of people receiving *private*
mental health care. For the benefit of patient and community, it

will be important for public and private sector care to influence each other. The challenge is to protect the financial integrity of the system while at the same time protecting clinical integrity.

In mental health care, there are now two sets of "customers." The first customers are the payers, public and private, who demand de-hospitalization. It is the payers who demand a hospital without walls. In fact, the continuum may best meet the needs of payers. The second customers are the patients or patients and their families. By providing options, this continuum may be meeting the needs of patients, but this has yet to be proven by research. We are not yet able to provide patients with the maximum benefit from the continuum concept. As physicians, we must consider the patients as our first customers.

The continuum is probably most problematic for the clinician. The clinician is now involved in a high-volume, high-turnover practice. Clinical decisions may be made without meeting the patient face-to-face. The clinician may find him- or herself traveling to different locations and bedeviled by unreimbursed services such as telephone calls and paperwork. Training young clinicians and retraining older ones is a crucial first step in deriving maximum benefit from the continuum.

This is a time of less money but more flexibility and more creativity. This is a time of experimentation and continuous quality improvement. Challenged by the demand for cost controls, clinical innovators must continue to learn how to do more with less.

Index

Page numbers printed in **boldface** type refer to tables or figures.

mentally ill–chemical abuse
  program, 105–106
  admission criteria for, 106
  therapeutic activities of,
    106
partial hospitalization,
  101–102
  admission to, 101
  discharge criteria for, 102
  length of stay in, 102
  objectives of, 101
  therapeutic activities of,
    101–102
range of, 92–94
Alcoholics Anonymous, 45, 94,
  100, 106, 194
*Allies and Adversaries: The
  Impact of Managed Care on
  Mental Health Services,* 1
Alzheimer's disease, 194–195,
  199–200
American Association for Partial
  Hospitalization, 157
Americans With Disabilities Act,
  348
Antabuse, 195
Antidepressants, 201, 239
Antipsychotics, 57, 116
Assaultive behavior, 196
Assertive community treatment
  teams, 29
Attention-deficit/hyperactivity
  disorder, 141, 334

Barriers to care, 5
Behavioral group practices,
  20–24
  administrative characteristics
    of, 21, 23–25

clinical characteristics of,
    22–23
  development and growth of,
    21
  independent practice
    associations, 21
  major challenges to, 24–25
  management service
    organizations and, 21
  networks of, 21–22
  patient access, intake, and
    triage in, 22
  structured as carve outs or
    carve ins, 20
Benefit-driven reimbursement
  system, 213–215
"Best practices" mandate, 238
Biopsychosocial treatment
  approach, 39, 93
Bipolar disorder, 239
  acute inpatient treatment for,
    110, 116
  case example of, 198–199
Brief focused psychotherapy,
  13–14, 305–306. *See also*
  Time-effective therapy
"Buddy" system, 72

Capitation financing, 2–4, 168
Caregivers for elderly patients,
  205–206
Carve outs and carve ins, 20
Case finding, 206–207
Case formulation, 236
Case management, 3, 7,
  218–219, 229–242
  for children, 334, 335
  clinical decision making and,
    230–234

child-foster parent
matching for, 136
patient population for,
132–133
respite care in, 137
selecting therapeutic foster
parents for, 133–135
supervision of, 136–137
training for, 135–136
in residential treatment
centers, 126–127,
131–132, 139–149
scope of, 125–126
in therapeutic foster homes,
129–130
Fountain House, 327
Fragmentation of services,
342–343, 360

Gatekeeper program, 207
Gatekeeping process, 5, 357
Global budgeting, 1, 4
Goal-oriented care, 5, 232–233
Goals of treatment, 236–237
Green Spring Health Services,
238
Group homes for children and
adolescents, 130
Group practices. *See* Behavioral
group practices
Group psychotherapy, 17

Halfway houses, 2, 61, 68–70.
See also Community
residential care for adults
Hallucinations, 115–116
High-intensity community
residences, 63–65
History taking, 235–236

Hobbies, 347–348
Home-based services (HBS), 2,
27–41. *See also* Positive
Alternatives to
Hospitalization program
and assessment of high-risk
cases, 35
benefits of, 40–41
case example of, 27–28
case management of, 29, 30,
37
characteristics of, 28–29
components critical to
success of, 39–40
accessible and available
care, 39
flexible, multimodal
approach, 39–40
least restrictive
environment, 39
patient's social support
system, 40
continuity of care maintained
by, 37
history of, 28
involvement of patient's
social support systems
in, 37
level of intensity of, 28, 36
outcomes research on, 38
treatment goals of, 35–38
crisis intervention, 36–37
patient and family risk
assessment, 35
quality improvement, 37–38
therapeutic alliance, 34–35
types of, 29–32, **30**
acute psychiatric crisis,
31–34

Panic disorder, 27, 271
Paranoia, 57
Parenting education, 30,
191–192
Parents, foster, 128–130,
133–135
Parsimony principle, 4, 14, 354
Partial hospital care programs,
2, 75–88
admission criteria for, 79, **80**
for alcohol and drug
treatment, 92, 94,
101–102
detoxification, 99–100
assessment and diagnosis in,
81–83
benefits of, **88**
case example of, 12, 75–77
census fluctuations in, 81
challenges and problems of,
88
for children and adolescents,
152–153
cost savings with, 217
definition of, 75
discharge criteria for, 79
discharge planning within,
79–81
facilities for, 86–87
physical plant
requirements, 86–87
sites, 86
functions of, 75
patient access to, 79
percentage of hospitals
offering, 217
referral to, 81
reimbursement for, **172**
staff roles in, 78

staff satisfaction with, 78
staffing patterns and ratios
for, 77–78
therapeutic activities of, 83–86
active therapies, 83
family involvement, 84
occupational
training/schooling, 84
program extenders, 84–85
special treatment
procedures and
emergency coverage,
85–86
therapeutic milieu, 83–84
unique aspects of, 87, **88**
PATHware, 248, 251–261, **255.**
See also Decision-support
software systems
patient risk mitigation
profile, **257**
patient risk severity profile,
256
patient risk severity scale, **258**
Patient advocacy, 29, 325, 333
Payers for care, 3, 19, 361
Personal dignity, 322
Personal interests of patients,
347–348
Personal psychotherapy for
psychiatric residents,
313–314
Personality disorders, 17, 34
*Persuasion and Healing: A
Comparative Study of
Psychotherapy,* 112–113
Pleasantville Cottage School,
127
Population-based perspective, 4,
14–15